Sue Matthews Petrovski

A
RETURN
JOURNEY

*Hope and Strength in the
Aftermath of Alzheimer's*

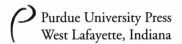

Purdue University Press
West Lafayette, Indiana

Library of Congress Cataloging-in-Publication Data

Petrovski, Sue Matthews.
   A return journey : hope and strength in the aftermath of Alzheimer's /
Sue Matthews Petrovski.
          p. cm.
Includes bibliographical references.
   ISBN 1-55753-302-4 (cloth: alk. paper)
   1. Alzheimer's disease—Patients—Home care. 2.   Caregivers.   I.
Title.
   RC523.P43 2003
   362.1'96831—dc21

2003007670

Do Not Go Gentle Into That Good Night

Do not go gentle into that good night,
Old age should burn and rave at close of day;
Rage, rage against the dying of the light.

Though wise men at their end know dark is right,
Because their words had forked no lightning they
Do not go gentle into that good night.

Good men, the last wave by, crying how bright
Their frail deeds might have danced in a green bay,
Rage, rage against the dying of the light.

Wild men who caught and sang the sun in flight,
And learn, too late, they grieved it on its way,
Do not go gentle into that good night.

Grave men, near death, who see with blinding sight
Blind eyes could blaze like meteors and be gay,
Rage, rage against the dying of the light.

And you, my father, there on the sad height,
Curse, bless me now with your fierce tears, I pray.
Do not go gentle into that good night.
Rage, rage against the dying of the light.

—Dylan Thomas,
from *The Poems of Dylan Thomas,*
copyright ©1952 by Dylan Thomas.
Reprinted with permission of
New Directions Publishing Corp.

To my mother and my father and all of those with
Alzheimer's Disease who have lived with delight
and "raged against the dying of the light."

Contents

Acknowledgements

What has a writer to be bombastic about?
Whatever good a man may write is the
consequence of accident, luck, or surprise,
and nobody is more surprised than an
honest writer when he makes a good
phrase or says something truthful.

—Edward Dahlburg

Dahlberg's comment celebrates and acknowledges the subjective nature of the written word, but he omits the fact that most ideas are generated in the collective mind and are only reworked or reorganized by the writer. No work about Alzheimer's caregivers can be complete without the contribution of many caring people; together we write these words, and together we fight this disease that causes us all so much pain.

My deepest admiration goes to those on the frontlines: the doctors, nurses, social workers, and other professionals who dedicate their lives to support those caught in the Alzheimer's trap, and to the researchers working conscientiously to add Alzheimer's to the list of diseases conquered. My gratitude goes to the following:

Tom Meuser, Ph.D. and director of Education and Rural Outreach, Alzheimer's Disease Research Center, Washington University, St. Louis; Ann Collins, R.N.; Geri Hall, Ph.D., College of Nursing and Behavioral Neurology, University of Iowa; Daniel L. Paris, MSW, CSW, formerly of Massachusetts General Hospital and currently with Cabrini Medical Center, New York, New York; Dr. Christopher Filley, University of Colorado School of Medicine; Whit Garberson, MSW, currently with the Massachusetts Department of Public Health, Special Needs Division; Dr. Eugene DuBoff, medical director of the Denver Center for Medical Research; Dr. Alan McCutcheon, M.D., specialist in geriatric medicine, Fremantle Hospital, Freemantle, Western Australia and honorary medical director of the Alzheimer's Association of Washington; Dr. Yuval Zabar, Boston; Lisa Gwyther, ACSW, Duke University; and many others. I thank you for your willingness to share your knowledge and the significant part each of you currently plays in educating caregivers and caring for the afflicted.

My thanks to all those caregivers who have communicated their feelings so unselfishly, and to the Alzheimer's patients who have shown a strength I wish I had. A special blessing to Carol, Cathy, Bud, Peter, and Martha. Without you, my earliest friends and co-caregivers, I would not have started this book. From you I gained a special understanding of this disease. A special thanks to Barbara Sorenson, my first interview. She so openly and frankly shared her feelings and story that it encouraged me to ask others for their story. Barbara, I will never forget the "Black Pill." Thanks to the caregivers who have given me permission to tell your stories, and to those who have asked that their names be omitted in order to keep their privacy. Readers should remember that for every story included in this manuscript, there are 10,000 more that need to be told.

Much of the caregiver information came, with each person's permission, from the online support group sponsored by the Alzheimer's Disease Research Center, Washington University, St. Louis. I thank them for giving me consent to use material from their site.

My deepest gratitude goes to Tamara Chapman for reading and editing the early drafts of this book and smoothly leading me to completion. Her gentle red reminders and intelligent ideas helped create some of the best parts of the book.

The support of Marcia Reish, Sharon Ramel, and the staff at the Rocky Mountain Chapter of the Alzheimer's Association has given me the confidence, the support, and the opportunity to work with caregivers in the Denver area. They have steadfastly encouraged me to continue working on the book, even when it seemed an impossible task. I have gained an understanding that I cannot begin to explain from my volunteer hours spent at our local chapter.

My thanks to Jean Boylan, director of the Rocky Mountain Chapter's "Memories in the Making" program, who has made it possible for art created in our local program to be a part of this book.

A special thanks to Mark Warner of Ageless Design (www.ageless design.com). A blessing on him for reading the rough copy and poking me every now and then to complete it. Thank you, Mark, for all you do for the Alzheimer's community, and for your encouragement and your kindness.

Thank you also to the staff at Purdue University Press for their invaluable help.

Lastly, I cherish the love of my family who continue to have confidence in my ability and suffered with me through the years of my mother's pain. My husband's kind spirit toward Mother and his willingness to support whatever had to be done to provide for her care was invaluable. He continues to believe in me and allow me to follow my dreams, sustaining me as I go. What do women do who don't have a husband they can confide in and trust to be there when times are tough? I don't know, because I do have such a husband. And to my writer-daughter Leslie, I thank you deeply for your ear and your advice. You will write the next book. And to Jon, my son: Whenever you were really needed you were there, and I can always depend on you for your intelligent opinions.

A Return Journey is a *fait accompli* because of all these friends and my dear family. By sharing and endowing me with their kindness and gracious support, as well as giving me pep talks when I lagged, they have made *A Return Journey* a book. Without them, it was only an experience.

—Sue Petrovski, June, 2003

A RETURN JOURNEY

Hope and Strength in the
Aftermath of Alzheimer's

PART ONE

CARING AND CAREGIVING

Introduction to Part One:
An Explanation of *A Return Journey*

> *The human heart dares not stay away*
> *from that which hurt it most.*
> *There is a return journey to anguish*
> *that few of us are released from making.*
> —Lillian Smith, *Killers of the Dream*

My mother's death was, at long last, a fact. We had survived eight years of the type of anguish that Lillian Smith suggests, and still my mind and heart refused to release the pain. What I had thought would be a time of intense relief, instead presented me with a whole new set of problems. Our long, painful trip through the twisted brainwaves of Mother's Alzheimer's disease had left me with little time for reflection. As is true of most caregivers, during her struggle I only seemed to have time to care for her pathetic physical needs, to make decisions that never seemed to be right, to cry, and to become more and more depressed by her unhappy existence. In short, I don't think I handled it well—I *know* I didn't handle it well—and at her death, a time of intense introspection overwhelmed me. Like so many caregivers I felt a welcome relief at the fact of death, but soon discovered it was a false lull. I had unexamined issues and pain that needed to be considered and dealt with. It was then that I began to mend.

Alzheimer's is a form of dementia. It traps its victims, inch by inch, in a time warp in which there are no yesterdays and no tomorrows, no familiar friends, no family, and no security beyond the moment. While it holds them there, it can cause the loved one to imagine all kinds of threatening delusions, like seeing things that aren't there and not being able to see that which is there. It can happen to us at age thirty, forty, and fifty, but more often at seventy or eighty. Whenever it strikes, from that moment on, that family is never the same.

Alzheimer's is a ravenous thief. It takes the personhood, the memories, the remembrances, and the sweet nature of the one we love. Before a fair share of a person's life is lived, that life is yanked away and secreted amid the tangles of mental confusion.

"I'm so alone," my mother would cry. "You say you're my daughter? Oh good! I didn't think I had any family."

This hurt worst of all. With every flicker of an eyelash, her world was lost forever, only to be replaced by an unknown world with unknown people. Minute by minute my mother, like all Alzheimer's patients, had to reinvent herself to fit into new, unknown surroundings inhabited by new and unknown persons. Without any understanding of what was really happening to her, we mouthed platitudes. "She really doesn't know what's happening, do you think?" Or, "People are more than their memories." Looking back, these mindless phrases sound so patronizing. "People are more than their memories." Long after the struggle was over, I realized the true significance of this particular platitude, but at the time it was only a form of mental pabulum I mouthed without thinking. Such trite phrases often become our survival techniques.

For eight years we watched as this dreadful disease transformed Mother into another person. We steadied her fears and studied her moods as best we could. We kept her physically safe, all of this exacting a tremendous mental and emotional toll. Then suddenly, Mother was gone. At her death, our friends and family encouraged me to forget past pain and move on. "Chin up!" "Keep a firm eye toward the future." "Buck up." "Don't give in to maudlin meanderings." "Get with it and get busy." I assured myself that they must be right. Two hundred million Americans can't be wrong. Hello, Sue, this is your culture talking.

At the risk of seeming whiny and immovable, I somehow knew it was healthier for me to return and deal with the demons that existed in the grief of those eight years. Then I could move on. We all want to obliterate pain, and we grasp at the sense of relief that death after such an ordeal seems to bring, but sometimes we avoid the reality of what we are really feeling. I call it the "empty hand" syndrome. When death finally arrives, a caregiver is left with the feeling of "What can I do now? I'm a caregiver, and I have been one for ___ years. Now I have no one to care for." In addition to the loss of the loved one, the caregiver must also deal with the loss of personal identity and purpose. Before I could go on, I had to find purpose. I had to find myself once again.

Another question that was important for me to consider was what rational significance, if any, Mother's years of pain and torment had served. Had Mother's life been wasted during those eight years? What meaning was there to her suffering? Was there any value to those smudged years or is life, after all, just a parade of meaningless, often painful, ups and downs?

Finally, it was for my own soul's sake that I needed time to make closure with this grotesque episode in our lives. I needed to mourn the loss of my mother and the part of myself that died with her. I needed to cry and get angry. I needed to kick things and rage to the heavens. Putting other important things on hold, I had to go back and remember. I had to make a return journey to that which came close to being my undoing. Why? Because of my deepest fears; no matter how it hurt, I had to make peace with those Alzheimer's ghosts, the phantoms of guilt and anger, the demons of depression and sorrow, the spirits that kept whispering, "Did you really do your best for your mother?" "Why weren't you there twenty-four hours a day, seven days a week for her?" "Couldn't you have cared for her at home until the end? How selfish you were!" Was I selfish? I had to find out. I could not live with the ambiguity.

And so I began to write. I began to reconstruct and rebuild the life that had been pulled down around me, hoping I could find an answer that I could live with. Feeling as though I was entering a burning building, I wrote about surviving; I wrote about depression, about the emotions I felt while caring for my demented mother; I wrote about grief as I was experiencing it and as I had experienced it every day for eight years. I investigated my love for my mother, going back well beyond the Alzheimer's years, and I tried to take an honest look at my own conduct, morality, and motivations during her illness.

For those who have tried it, you know that objectivity isn't easy. For two years following my mother's death, I viewed the final period of her life through half-closed, self-serving eyes. I suppose I was trying to shield my soul and conscience from painful truths. It was excruciating to look at what I considered my stupid and thoughtless mistakes, but I had no other choice. *I had to hold this ball of grief in my hand, examine it, and award it whatever rational significance it deserved before I could go on with my life.*

Note, I said *rational significance.* Obviously, we can feel pain forever if we continue to ball up emotionally every time we think of past grief. Somehow, I had to find a way to reach forward while still looking backward. How was I to heal? For me, the mending began when I started my return journey into the flames, into the pain: feeling the hurt, admitting the sorrow, and letting others know how badly I was scarred. It helped me to discuss it again and again, to write about it until the scar tissue thickened. Mother has been dead for several years. I never healed, but I mended.

This book became my flight plan to mental health. It started as a catharsis for my own healing. I wrote essays, I journaled, I posted e-mail messages to fellow caregivers. I collected sad and funny stories from my caregiver friends. Gradually, I discovered that I wasn't traveling alone. There are a lot of us out there—those whose scars never quite heal. We walk around with open wounds that no one can see. We hurt, but those around us are unaware of our pain.

Most of us expected to experience relief once the suffering of our loved ones had ended, but we found instead that we were left with Alzheimer's baggage that we might never shed. After steadfastly focusing on the disease which had consumed so much of our lives, we found ourselves unable to push on to other concerns. We were in the Alzheimer's cul-de-sac: arms empty, loved one gone, and a pain so deep we could only just barely touch it.

Losing a loved one to Alzheimer's or any other dementia is like no other loss. I lost a father to cancer, yet I could talk to him until the day he died. We could love and connect. He acted in a rational manner and, in his strong way, led us to a beautiful conclusion to his life. Alzheimer's isn't like that. It's a messy disease. Pain, anger, paranoia, hallucinations, cutting words, and our sins of omission and frustration leave wounds and sometimes cause permanent scars.

The result of my return journey was that I *literarily* mourned my mother. Bit by bit, journal entry by journal entry, I began putting the pieces of my grief together; these scraps of consciousness became *A Re-*

turn Journey. As I wrote, I developed a group of friends on the Internet and at our local Alzheimer's Association. I had become wise enough to discover my need for others, and I finally understood the fact that I could not repair myself all by myself. It was a reassurance to discover that other caregivers had experienced the same demons and ghosts and were willing to help console me in my grief.

A Return Journey is not about physical caregiving. Put this book down now if you want to learn how to safeguard your loved one from wandering or kitchen dangers. Don't look here for advice on choosing a doctor. Many excellent resources can help you with these concerns. Although *A Return Journey* shares stories about the common problems of caregiving, it focuses on the challenges and attitudes—grief, guilt, anger, love, and hate—experienced by caregivers. It's those things that drive us to examine our own worth. It is also those things that help us survive. It is about coping.

In *A Return Journey,* Alzheimer's caregivers have shared very personal letters, journal entries, essays, and notes. Better than anything, these illustrate how we felt when each day was a battleground bringing yet another new problem. In these scraps from the past, we confess to the anger that arises when our loved ones ask the same question over and over all day long. We explain how each day is a death of some precious part of our loved one, eaten up inch by inch, word by word, by the enemy who always wins. Grandchildren, daughters, sons, husbands, and wives have said, "Please look at our pain. Look at this tragedy. Look at what we have learned, and look at how we grew stronger." My friend, Michele, says it so well:

> Yesterday I was thinking that as horrible as this disease is, it has somehow made ME a better person. I am so much more compassionate. I have learned to show love when I felt none or little was shown to me for so very long. I have learned to hug, even though I can't remember getting one since I was a child. I have learned to empathize with the confusion and pain that my mother is feeling and to give my all to calm those anxieties. And I have learned to feel the depth of my soul, which was hidden away for so very long. So, in this particular case, the disease is not claiming two victims, but it has actually made one of us a better human being.

We hope we have avoided the temptation to lecture, to complain, or to generalize beyond the point of usefulness. We share our experiences in hopes that those who have never experienced Alzheimer's will better understand its complexity and that those who are presently coping will know they are not alone. Let us not permit this terrible disease any more victims than necessary.

The author dedicates any profits from this book to Alzheimer's education and research.

ONE
The Enormity of It All

C. has small children and normally she maintains a "steady as you go" lifestyle. Few things shock her. There is little that sends her into depression or anxiety. Reluctantly, she reveals her uncharacteristic reaction to her father's new illness:

> When I take off all my facades and expose my vulnerable self, I am a little girl who is watching her daddy disappear brain cell by brain cell. I feel alone, frightened, sad, and very overwhelmed.
>
> I would rather I had lost my left arm than have to watch my dad, this brilliant man with an advanced degree, a man I have always looked up to, a very prideful man, reduced to a shell of nothingness. Now I have to talk to him like I talk to my two-year-old.

The anger and frustration that comes hand in hand with grief can be heard when C. adds:

> I've had it with reality; I want a fairy godmother! I hate watching my mom's "happily ever after" turned into this twisted disease. I don't want my dad to die like this! Anybody got a magic pill? I seem to have misplaced my magic wand.

Alzheimer's is an enormous illness. Little by little a beloved person is lost to a disease that seems to use some mental slight of hand, magically replacing him or her with a stranger. The non-involved see our loved ones as no more than pathetically-addled beings. They never comprehend the reality of the transition from a fully functioning individual to an Alzheimer's patient. The uninitiated cannot begin to understand what we experience. As we watch our loved ones disintegrate, we madly try to adjust medications, invent cures, and provide needed care for whatever the disease leaves on our doorstep. Our total being is focused on just one more day of keeping our person with us.

Charlotte lives in Seattle. Her mother died in November 2000, but, "she was showing signs of the disease much, much earlier." She explains why Alzheimer's is so terrible:

> There are chronic conditions like epilepsy and diabetes, chronic depression, and arthritis that we just learn to live with, and part of living with them is managing them and controlling them. You have some control over these conditions. Not that it's easy, for these diseases are an added challenge to life. But *we* are in charge, even though they are, for the most part, incurable.
>
> But there are conditions that you can't just learn to live with. These are the conditions you must learn to die with. They can't be treated and they can't be cured. The symptoms can't even be managed effectively for very long. My father has one of those conditions called Primary Schleroscing Chlangitis (PSC). It's a liver disease, and you can't do anything for it at all except put your name on the transplant list and hope you get a new liver before you die.
>
> However, when people are diagnosed with this sort of disease they don't have to despair. They can take charge of what's left of their living and of their dying. They can give it meaning, and they can die well. But Alzheimer's is a truly horrible disease because it robs you of your ability to learn. As a result, you can't learn how to live with the disease and you can't learn how to die with it. It robs you of the ability to die well. It robs you of the peace and dignity and even the joy that comes with working through your diagnosis, of accepting it, of coming to terms with your mortality, of making peace with those you love, and of making plans for your own death.

How terribly sad.

In addition to the grief we feel for our loved one, we flinch every time they let us see the confusion and frustration they are feeling. Sally shares this:

> Mother's not sleeping as much. She sees furniture from her mother's house and wonders how it got here. Then she gets upset when she doesn't know something she thinks she should know and says, "I'm crazy. I'm nuts. I'm cuckoo." She doesn't always know that I'm her daughter, although she does know I care for her, that she lives with me and my family, and that I tell her I love her every

night when she goes to bed. She was panicky over the weekend about not knowing how all this "stuff" (furniture from her parents' house) had gotten here, where "here" *is*, and so on.

Much like an alien form that assumes many shapes, Alzheimer's is a complex conundrum of symptoms admitting to no fixed solution. Alzheimer's patients exhibit memory problems. This is a given. However, with Alzheimer's, the forgetting may be of entire experiences. This is joined with a gradual inability to follow written or spoken directions. Notes soon become an ineffective tool, and patients become unable to care for themselves. However, in Mild Cognitive Impairment, or MCI, a term reserved for those with only memory loss, parts of an experience are forgotten and may soon be remembered. They are usually able to use notes as mental aids and can usually care for themselves (Overview of Alzheimer's Disease and Related Disorders 4–5).

Losses in these areas bring about needs that the caregiver has to supply. If they are not supplied, the result is unwanted, needs-driven behavior. In the early stages, a loved one may be able to discuss the weather and world events but not know how to write a check. This may cause great anxiety and frustration. He or she may be able to enjoy dinner and a movie, but not know what a theater ticket is for. The resulting behavior may be irrational and angry.

We know that what works today may not work tomorrow, and what works for one person may not work for another. Without any preparation or training, we are required to communicate with a nonreasoning human being. *How long will it last? When will it end? Does this thing just keep getting worse and worse? Why does he seem to hate me?*

Yet we continue to push ourselves, exercising our loved ones and massaging their tormented bodies. Frantically we search for obscure medical practitioners, lotions, ointments, and restoratives that will, perhaps, keep them alert for a tiny bit longer. We hate the reality of our loved ones' lives, yet we cannot come to grips with their deaths. We pray for a moment of sanity, a second of reality, a modicum of recognition, adjusting to whatever the split-second mood or need happens to be. Eventually, our only choice is to enter their reality because they have left our rational world.

A stranger we may secretly resent, want to avoid, and cannot begin to understand sits in front of us in need of care, and we aren't sure we are capable or willing to give it. Frankly, there often seems little to love about the Alzheimer's person—a person who is confused, fearful, paranoid, this *someone* who may scream, swear, and be unaware of the niceties of life, this *someone* with a hunted, wild, fearful look in the eye. Day by day we pray for a scrap of evidence that our person is there: a smile, a look, a familiar phrase, a tiny joke. As the disease progresses, Alzheimer's caregivers ask for very little.

As Alzheimer's nibbles through the brain selectively choosing different paths for each person, it is difficult to predict what ability it will attack next. Experienced caregivers warn us, "If you know one Alzheimer's patient, you know one Alzheimer's patient." Even though no typical scenario characterizes Alzheimer's, it does involve a series of symptoms in pattern-like form.

An All-Too-Familiar Scenario

Let us suppose that a hypothetical mother, loved by her family, is beginning to do things that are dangerous to her safety. She forgets appointments, doesn't take medications as directed, and sometimes lets strangers into the house when it could be inappropriate. Perhaps she is doing strange things to her checking account, or she may be buying too many Lotto tickets. The family begins to notice changes in her verbal patterns. She grasps for words, often coming up with gibberish and getting frustrated when she cannot find the word she is searching for. Typically, these changes come on gradually and get more pronounced with time. Never fear, Alzheimer's *is* progressive. The family will soon see the entire picture.

The family wants to get help in the home, someone to help care for their mother. By this time she may be refusing to bathe or brush her teeth, or she may be trying to wear three sweaters or four pairs of panties. The mother may be collecting all sorts of trash: plastic bags and containers, old food cartons, outdated magazines, or last year's newspapers. A visit to her home may be like a trip to the city dump. Food in the refrigerator may be moldy or spoiled, yet the mother becomes more and more stubborn, flatly refusing any help. She is apt to say, "I've always done for myself, and I can do so now."

It is likely that she has some idea of what's happening to her and is hoping that, by retreating into an ever-tightening world, she can protect herself from exposure. She is afraid. Typically, the family is hesitant to override a mother's will. After all, they have listened to her give directions all their lives, and the idea of *telling* Mom anything is thorny, particularly since most families are unsure of what to do themselves. Even a spouse will try desperately to heed the wishes of a demented mate, carrying on a loving habit of many shared years.

Our hypothetical mother begins to get nervous and anxious, often in the late afternoon. This is called *sundowning*. For some reason, maybe fatigue, the four o'clock witching hour can bring out the worst in Alzheimer's patients. They can hallucinate, become totally confused, and be very difficult to live with. Mother may become paranoid, suspecting family members of stealing from her. She accuses and berates those closest to her. She may have a fetish about her pocketbook, which she loses fifty times a day and accuses family members of taking. She may begin to wander or get lost, and if pushed into a corner of fear, she may lash out. She may insist that men have come into her home and robbed her.

If the family honestly looks at the situation, chances are they will find she is having difficulty with many daily activities. She is no longer safe around a stove, and a check on her medications indicates they are not being taken properly. Care must be taken to keep her from leaving home. If she drives a car, eventually she *must* be stopped. In a later stage, she becomes incontinent and gradually begins to forget even her own children or husband. Finally, she is unable to identify herself. Her memories of her childhood seem like today to her, while today has yet to happen. She is alone in a demented mind in a friendless world.

The family looks for answers. "Let's try a change of medication." Arguments may ensue about what constitutes the best care for the mother. Who will take her into their home? "Perhaps we should consider an assisted-living facility. How about a nursing home?" Some family members feel that mountains are being made of molehills. "Grandma is an adult. Let her do as she wishes. She's just getting senile." Senile means aged and, contrary to popular opinion, dementia is not a natural part of aging. And the most serious question is, "How can we keep her safe?" This is usually followed by a more difficult question. "How can we make her happy?" Safe, maybe. Happy might be a long shot.

Mental Chaos

When facing a difficult task, act as
though it is impossible to fail.
If you're going after Moby Dick,
take along the tarter sauce.

—Anonymous

If I want to conquer this disease, it becomes clear that I must have more ammunition. First, I need to know more about what Alzheimer's actually does to the brain. Dr. Christopher M. Filley, professor of neurology and psychiatry at the University of Colorado School of Medicine, explains it as well as it can be explained:

> Many disorders of the brain, and AD in particular, involve the erosion of the fundamental qualities by which we define our existence. In short, it gradually destroys consciousness, that fundamental quality of human existence.
> Research now indicates that the disease process—neuritic plaques, neurofibrillary tangles, loss of synapses, and neuronal death —occurs first and most prominently in the areas of the brain that are the most recent to appear in development. In other words, the disease selectively attacks those uniquely human skills that evolution has so carefully produced over millions of years.
> The exquisite order of the brain, the most vital key to our adaptive success, is assaulted and mental chaos results (Filley 4–5).

Mental chaos. Few of us can comprehend the gigantic tasks accomplished by our brains. We aren't able to speak, think, love, feel, chew, walk, swallow, or create without the brain. We can't even scratch our head. Alzheimer's cannot be reasoned away because there is no reason left. Reason flies out the window the moment Alzheimer's flies in. The word dementia comes from "de" in Latin, meaning "away from" and "mens," which in Latin, interestingly enough, can mean "mind, intellect, judgment, feelings, disposition, courage, opinion, thoughts, intention, or resolve." We have to remember that dementia means "out of mind." Think about it. Alzheimer's dementia is not *only* a loss of memory. It is a loss of *all* of the mental attributes: intellect, judgment, disposition, opinion, and resolve. *It is a loss of personhood.*

A State of Shock

There has not been enough information in the media to make the public knowledgeable about Alzheimer's disease, but there has been just enough to cause dreadful fear. The first thing to remember about Alzheimer's is that the diagnosis of a loved one is usually a horror to the family. We don't know what we fear, but we know enough to know it can't be good. For this and other reasons, doctors are cautious and hesitant about making the final diagnosis.

At present, autopsy is the only sure means of diagnosis. Our current diagnostic procedures are basically a process of elimination. Eliminate all other possible causes for the condition and we are left with *probable Alzheimer's*. I have heard many caregivers say, "Well, they're not sure it's Alzheimer's." The doctor said, "It's only *probable Alzheimer's*." Well, that's as good as it gets at the present time. We are just beginning to scratch the surface of more subtle diagnoses, and some researchers are even beginning to question whether early-onset Alzheimer's[1] is really Alzheimer's. Be that as it may, even with even more sophisticated tools, we have to be very careful of our diagnosis. Dr. Alan McCutcheon, staff specialist in geriatric medicine at Fremantle Hospital says:

> There isn't a scan that can diagnose AD. How could it when the diagnosis depends on the microscopic appearance of the individual cells? CT scans can show the general structure of the brain, MRI scans can distinguish more efficiently between different types of tissue, SPECT scans can show circulation patterns, PET scans can show metabolic patterns, but to make the diagnosis of AD for sure you need some of the brain tissue under a microscope.
>
> It certainly can help if you have a clinical story consistent with AD and the SPECT scan shows reduced perfusion (circulation) to medial temporal and posterior parietal lobes. That is a typical pattern for AD, but doesn't make the diagnosis.

Knowing how the term Alzheimer's can panic families and being, perhaps, a bit unsure of a questionable diagnosis, doctors may use the general term *dementia*. Other times they may resort to the old-fashioned term, *senile dementia,* and I've even heard the term *chronic brain syndrome* used, whatever that is. Sometimes a complete diagnosis may take months as doctors rule out all possible causes and wait to see if the condition is progressive. We want them to be careful, for an Alzheimer's diagnosis is not a diagnosis that is easy to come to terms with. It is a diagnosis that must be made with great care.

Soon after a family gets the Alzheimer's word they will probably enter a state of shock. "It must be wrong, let's get another diagnosis. Well, she's not that bad yet!" Denial rears its dangerous head. It influences us to under- or overmedicate, turn a blind eye to strange and unsettling living conditions, and allow unsupervised and dangerous activities. A refusal to face what is happening causes us to avoid taking a strong stand on issues such as driving or wandering and generally avoid financial, legal, and health matters that should be handled before the disease progresses too far.

All too often, close family members say something like, "I just don't understand this thing at all. She's fine, usually. She can cook okay and dresses herself. It's just *some* things she has trouble with." Nothing wrong with this is there? No, except that it becomes a logical next step to say, "Well, if she can cook, why did she act so stupid yesterday and not know a tablespoon from a teaspoon? Maybe she's just being stubborn." We desperately try to catch our loved ones in time and clutch at the idea that this is as bad as it will get or that perhaps they're only pretending. No. If it is Alzheimer's, it will only progress onward.

Fog

The fog comes
On little cat feet
It sits looking
Over harbor and city
On silent haunches
And then moves on.

—Carl Sandburg,
from *Chicago Poems.* Reprinted
in cooperation with Dover Publications.

An added burden is the fact that, at present, we are unable to "fix" Alzheimer's. Our western culture, which prescribes, describes, designs, and fixes, collapses on us when unable to put it right. How does a rational culture deal with irrationality? Poorly. If not prepared for Alzheimer's ambiguities, caregivers can suffocate and die in the process of trying to cope with the disease.

The effective Alzheimer's doctor must deal with the family as well as the patient. But at times, although they can diagnose and prescribe, medical staff often seem to deny responsibility for helping a family with suggestions for day-to-day care. A survey by the Alzheimer's Association found that only thirty-one percent of caregivers believe that their doctors were of help in finding services, while ninety-seven percent of doctors said they had given such advice. ("Survey Finds Large Communication Gap Between Doctors and Alzheimer's Caregivers," 1)

Orien Reid, chair of the association's national board of directors and a former caregiver, frankly says:

> Alzheimer's caregiving is particularly hard work, and caregivers face enormous physical and emotional stresses in taking care of their loved ones. Caregivers need information and support to cope with this devastating disease. Not having all the information they need decreases their ability to make sure family members are receiving the most effective treatment and care and increases their guilt and frustration as they try to figure out how to cope with the disease (Reid 1).

Although support is much easier to find today than ten years ago, aside from the Alzheimer's Association, institutionalized sources are still minimally supportive. Nursing homes and assisted-care facilities may advertise that they are Alzheimer's proficient but may be unwilling to accept any patient with a history of aggressiveness. Care for the difficult patient is hard to locate. Caregivers, with even less training than the professionals, are then left alone to deal with the wildest of behaviors while trying desperately to find a safe refuge for their loved one. Add to that the present difficulty in finding qualified personnel in all areas of health care, and we can begin to see the wide gaps in the quality of care available.

Our government, which provides equipment and residential care for many illnesses through the Medicare program, panics at the thought of providing the kind of care that Alzheimer's patients need. The fear of getting involved in an expensive caregiving disease scares away tax dollars that could give caregivers tremendous support. When they get together to chat, many families confess that once Alzheimer's came into their lives, their friends and their government were the last to offer help. Forced to use life savings in order to care for their loved one, they honestly feel like they have the plague. Why? Because that is how our culture sees Alzheimer's: as a plague, an expensive plague.

An Ohio State University study showed that caring for a family member with Alzheimer's exacts a steep emotional and physical toll on the caregiver. In fact, stress for caregivers appears to be long-term, lingering for at least two years after the death of the Alzheimer's patient. This study of sixty-two caregivers compared the psychological states and the immune functions of current caregivers to those whose loved ones died two years previously. Both groups were matched against a control group of men and women with no caregiving experience.

The researchers found that those presently caring for family members with Alzheimer's, and those who had cared for a loved one with Alzheimer's in the past showed identical levels of depression and stress. Both groups experienced significantly more depression and stress than the non-caregivers. Caregivers also displayed decreased immune system responses as measured by natural killer (NK) cell activity. NK cells are a special class of white blood cells that find and destroy tumor cells and other invaders such as viruses (Squires z5).

These findings could explain why caregivers report having more colds, flu, and other respiratory illnesses than other segments of the population. One theory attributes this to the fact that caregivers often are elderly themselves and their immune systems may have more difficulty recovering from stress.

A CNN report by Elizabeth Cohen examined a study comparing stress on the body's immune system from various sources including bad traffic, muggings, marriage problems, and caring for a spouse with Alzheimer's. Researchers ranked the sources according to long-term adverse effects on the immune system. Psychologist Janice Kiecolt-Glaser found that a bad marriage and caring for an Alzheimer's spouse tied for the worst health hazards.

This report also found that people under constant stress, such as caregivers, have twice the cancer rate of those without these stresses as well as an increased risk for heart attacks and high blood pressure. One conclusion drawn is that the way to help fight stress was to "let go, or get help." (CNN.com).

Alzheimer's is a difficult thing to simply "let go." So the answer is to "get help." Somehow, this is often the hardest thing to do. Recently a caregiver in poor health and in his eighties was sobbing because he could not care for his wife at home. Total in-home care could cost him over $80,000 a year. He will be forced to place her in a nursing home and even then the cost would be about $50,000 a year or more.

Facts and Figures

Current estimates indicate that approximately four million Americans have Alzheimer's Disease. This suggests that nineteen million Americans have a family member with Alzheimer's and thirty-seven million know someone with the disease. The Alzheimer's Association estimates that *fourteen million* Americans will have Alzheimer's by 2050 and *twenty-two million* persons worldwide will be its victims by 2025.

Alzheimer's costs Americans at least $100 billion a year. Neither Medicare nor private health insurance covers the type of long-term care most patients need. Assisted living can cost families $2,500 to $8,000 a month. In many cases, neither Medicare or Medicaid[2] will pay for care in assisted-living sites, nor will Medicare pay for long-term care for Alzheimer's patients in nursing homes. If a family is not eligible for Medicaid, they may have to declare bankruptcy or sell their homes to pay expenses that are not covered. A nursing home today can cost $42,000 per year, exceeding $70,000 in some areas. Alzheimer's costs American businesses $33 billion annually, but most of this loss is not in direct care to patients. Most of it, $26.5 billion, is to lost productivity of caregivers and the rest is the business share in costs for health and long-term care (General Statistics/Demographics).

It helps me to understand the enormity of Alzheimer's when I consider that in Colorado we have more than 60,000 Alzheimer's patients. Our local baseball stadium, Coors Field, holds around 50,000 people.

Think of a huge stadium in every middle-to-large-sized American city spilling over with dementia patients and you get some feeling for our present circumstances. Even this graphic illustration doesn't begin to help us grasp the enormity of our future challenges, unless we accept Alzheimer's as a major world problem and mobilize for a war on this disease.

Caregivers can probably expect little help from the government and many have mixed feelings about the care provided at assisted-living facilities and nursing homes. Aside from the financial and housing problems that exist in dealing with Alzheimer's, I found the most destructive thing to me was the personal loss. How can we find help for that? C., who wanted a fairy godmother to take away the pain, is obviously aware of the disease in terms of tragic numbers, but to her, it is extremely personal. Statistics cannot describe what her family is going through. "I am just a little girl watching my daddy disappear brain cell by brain cell," she says. That's her reality.

We weep for our private wounds and ache for the pain suffered by our loved ones. Carla has been an Alzheimer's caregiver to her father for many years and is determined to wage a mighty battle, but where can she go for help when her father asks, "My mother is dead, isn't she?" Carla says:

> And I was caught in that moment, unable to lie. There seems a vast difference between accepting someone's delusion and creating one. His mother had been dead for twenty-five years. And I said, "Yes, Dad, she is."
>
> He wept because his mother had died. Another curse for the disease that makes present joys evaporate in minutes, and brings long-gone pains to the present to be lived again.

Alzheimer's is a cursed disease, causing our loved ones to endure pain over and over again while preventing them from recognizing the joys of the present. It erases a lifetime of memories and drains life savings. It requires minute-to-minute solutions to unsolvable problems, and caregivers have to watch it all happen, day after day, assured that nobody out there really cares.

A Return Journey's Message

So, is there any tarter sauce that will comfort the Alzheimer's person and assist families as they try to mentally and physically care for their loved ones? The Alzheimer's patient ultimately will not survive. The average lifespan today is eight to ten years from diagnosis with symptoms that are sometimes identifiable for as many as twenty years before that. (Facts: About Alzheimer's Disease). Caregivers may come away from the disease as walking wounded unless they are lucky enough to find a lifeline to clutch. Unfortunately, all too many caregivers burrow into the necessary caregiving and are swallowed up in the concerns of the moment. Their own physical and mental health simply takes a backseat. (See Appendix B: Caregivers Self-rating Scale.)

Looking back, I recognize my mistake in not taking the time to learn more about the disease and to communicate with others enduring the same circumstances. My choice was to "get on with it." Sadly, I paid for my blindness. Alzheimer's always wins, but I almost let it take two lives. I was too inexperienced to know how important attitude, education, and support were to my well-being and to the care of my mother. There were at least partial answers there in front of me, but I ignored them. I should have said, as Michele did in the introduction, "the disease is not claiming two victims."

When I was a child in southern Indiana, a storm would sometimes roll through the sky at a terrific, frightening speed. Dark and malignant, it would spin across the countryside, promising death and destruction. To a small child, the most frightening thing was the feeling of powerlessness. I felt lost in the storm's magnitude, chained to endure whatever destruction it willed.

Alzheimer's is like that. Make no mistake, it will take its course, no matter what you or I may do. It leaves us powerless but desperate for control. It causes us to run in circles thinking we might escape its wrath. It causes us to rationalize and deny what we see happening before us. Like a devil in disguise, Alzheimer's can tear away our spiritual supports and bring us to an anger we never knew we could feel. At present, shelter from its magnitude is woefully lacking. If *A Return Journey* can help us tunnel through our personal and social confusion to a place that is rational and whole, if after this experience we can say we are no longer as afraid, then it has been a useful mender.

> *In the dark times, will there also be singing?*
> *Yes, there will be singing, about the dark times.*
> —Bertolt Brecht

TWO
My Mother's Story

Mark Twain spoke of his daughter's death as something akin to a dreadful blaze that destroys one's home. Everything is lost, but it is only later, when time jogs us, that we appreciate the total extent of the irreplaceable riches we have lost. A person is *one of a kind* and can never be replaced. The heart mends, but it never completely heals.

My person was *one of a kind*. She could not be replaced. Much of the pain I felt at Mother's loss was the inner aching that comes from missing the essentials, the idiosyncrasies that define the one lost. We secretly know these essentials are irretrievable, and yet we return again and again to that burning house as though mesmerized. As we do, we discover more about ourselves and learn to manage the magnitude of our personal disaster.

It has been over six years since my mother's death from Alzheimer's, and I still find myself turning to tell her something or to ask her a question that only she can answer. I am still shocked when I realize she isn't there. Louisa May Alcott wrote, "What do girls do who haven't any mothers to help them through their troubles?" I don't know, because I had such a mother. And then the time came for me to help her through *her* final trouble. A small payment for what I had received from her, and yet I wondered if I had let her down.

Because Mother is the reason this book was written, I saved one chapter to tell you about her. This is it. In the following poem, "The Swing is Still," I returned to the burning house to discover the mother who cuddled me when I was a tiny child. Following that, I try to share the path on which that person I called Mother changed into someone I didn't know. Share the smoking wreckage with me:

The Swing is Still

"Oh how I love
To go up in a swing,
Up in the air so high.
Oh, I do think it's
The most wondrous thing . . . "

You were my beautiful mother,
Chattering and crooning to me,
"Just Molly and Me, and Baby Makes Three,
We're Happy in My Blue Heaven."

My Blue Heaven was there.
The creaking of the old green swing,
Hanging securely from the porch ceiling
Of our early home
Was accented by my frequent questions,
"Who's the baby?" I asked. But I knew.
"Why it is you." I loved to hear her say it.
"You are my baby, my darling child."
And I would curl my small bare toes
And wiggle with delight.

The summer stickiness of southern Indiana
Was always relieved by the sway of that swing
And the lilt of the poems
The two of us shared.
Our world was wrapped and entwined with our love.
While you shelled peas or mated socks,
The task at hand
Merging in my memory with the
Closeness, the dampness and the love.

"Do you remember 'The Little Shadow'?"
"I have a little shadow who goes in and out with me,
And what can be the use of him is more than I can see."
"Do you remember that?" You would ask.
Of course I did.
We had crooned it to one another over and over.

We both loved that little shadow
And as we said the precious words,
I sank closer to you,
Pushing the swing to chase away the scarier shadows
That lurked somewhere in the night.

But then the swing was still,
The tables turned,
And the shadows were not poetic, nor friendly.
The shadows of your illness
Lengthened our pain
And shortened the days of your life.

We abide in your illness, holding hands and crying,
And when I ask you why you cry, you shake your head and sigh.
When you ask me why the tears stream down my face,
I try to smile and say, "Oh, no reason. Just 'cause."
Unspoken, not acknowledged,
Your withering brain and unkempt gray locks
Doomed the halcyon days we had shared.

The arc of the swing slowed almost to a halt.
I had become the mother of my mother.
As Alzheimer's deepened and robbed her of her selfhood,
As the shadow of its destruction
Grew and grew,
My tongue was mute.
The pain of her pain made songs and games
And poets' lyrics dry in my mouth.
I could but cry for the grief I felt.

If once again we meet
In some far distant heaven,
I will ask your forgiveness,
Dear Mother of mine.
You nurtured me when I was small and insecure,
And taught me laughter and gay tunes.
The warmth of your bosom
And the nurture of your soul
Were there for me, unquestioned and serene.

But when you retreated,
Meeting your childhood long before your time,
When you needed me
I could not match the mother you had been.
I could not go into your childhood with you.

We could have swung on the swing so high,
As I hugged you in my arms.
We could have played
With clover blossoms,
And tied them into chains
For your ageless crown.

We could have whistled our tunes
On crab grass spikes,
Matching whatever age you wanted to be,
But we didn't, and I didn't,
And the swing has stopped.

Alas, as you became smaller,
And more in need,
As you became the child needing solace,
Frightened
And unknowing,
I could offer you no songs, no poetry.
I could naught but cry.

—Sue Petrovski

I could naught but cry. I wish I may, I wish I might . . . I wish I had been strong enough to hold my mother and laugh and play with her in her last childhood. Instead, the pain engulfed me. The stress of the disease made it impossible for me to relax and laugh with her in her final years. Because I was so tense, I only seemed to make her stress worse. Like a new-made mother, I stewed and wrung my hands and felt that Fate had landed *me* a cruel blow. I am sad to say that I was more concerned with my position than with the harshness of the blow dealt my mother.

I was the only child of Depression-era parents who had grown up in rural poverty. As such, I was sheltered and cared for as only that generation of Americans knew how to do it. I wasn't given a lot of material things, but my world was very secure. I was so sure of love, so sure of acceptance. Mother and Dad would say, "We're three bugs under a rug." I had many friends with whom I played kick the can and paper dolls, roller skated, and dressed up, but when I went home it was always "three bugs."

And then there were two bugs. Father died of cancer in the late eighties, leaving Mother and me feeling a great loss. The Bushmen of the Kalahari Desert believe it to be of major importance for the shaman to recite the correct incantations whenever a large animal is killed. They fear that if the ritual is not followed, great evil will enter the world and inhabit the enormous vacuum left by the animal's passing. I have sometimes wondered if the illness Mother suffered didn't enter at my father's death in some half-understood way. For both of us his death was a huge loss, but for her it was devastating.

Mother was the best playmate I ever had, but when problems arose we both turned to my father. His strength allowed her to play the child bride, and at his death something flickered out in her spirit. Her sense of humor and bright smiles soon were replaced by a tight, almost plastic persona given to minimal responses until, gradually, she became increasingly aloof, distant, and angry. Hugs were met with stiffness and most conversations with a dreamy, half-aware, "Hmmm, well, well." It was exactly like hitting a brick wall. Her stories disappeared. No more thoughtful presents for the grandchildren. No chitchat with neighbors. She read less and less and found TV an irritation more than an enjoyment. I waited in vain for a hug or a kiss or a smile of recognition. One bug was gone and one was obviously badly damaged. Not knowing what was happening to my mother, I took her distant attitude at face value and backed into my own world.

And then it happened. It was Christmas night in 1989. Our adult children had long since grown tired of the celebration and left for their own homes. I sat in my office typing some thoughts to use the following week in my classroom. Mother lived with us in her own downstairs apartment. We had already noticed a tendency for her to forget to take medicines, lose her wayward purse, and repeat herself fifty times. But these were small, insignificant things we passed off as signs of aging. How many of us have done this?

My mind was occupied, and I scarcely heard the words that were to foretell the worst experience of our lives:

"Sue, isn't it time we went home? I don't know how to get there."
"What did you say, Mom?" Still I didn't grasp her words.
Her face was anxious, and she licked her lips and wrung her hands.
Again she said, "How do I get home? Aren't we going to leave soon?" I knew, at that moment, that this wasn't her usual forgetfulness.
"But, Mom, you are home. Don't you remember? We live here and you live downstairs."
"But how . . . where . . . I don't know . . . "

She was terribly confused, and I could tell that the confusion frightened her. I led her down to her apartment. As soon as she saw her own belongings she seemed relieved, secure and content at the sight of the familiar. Thus, for the moment, life continued. Little had changed, yet everything had changed. In that fleeting moment, my mother, with the file-cabinet mind, had not been able to find her way downstairs.

Alarm number one had sounded, and acknowledging that we had a problem catapulted me from one realm of reality into another. Leaving the kingdom of the so-called rational, we had to adjust to a maelstrom of the irrational. In a flea-flick of time, the world was upside down. It was impossible on that hallowed Christmas night to conceive of the change that was about to occur in our lives. At first, we chalked the experience up to fatigue, shutting out the nagging non-sequiturs, sure that this would probably never happen again. How wrong we were.

Early on, my conversations with Mother consisted of her asking the same question over and over and me answering over and over, until I inevitably would flare up in anger. If I became annoyed enough, she would leave me alone for a while, but my anger left me with a load of guilt that didn't solve the looming questions that were mounting day by day.

When dementia enters a family, everyone's role is suddenly and irrevocably altered. If it happens to your parent or spouse, you become the parent. Never again will the world look quite as it did. Never again will you be assured of your sanity, for to enter the world of the demented we must accept the realities of that confused world and work within its undefined and tricky boundaries. My confidence in myself as a caregiver was miniscule and so was my knowledge of the disease. I dreaded, loathed, and avoided the multitude of challenges, questions, conditions, personality changes, and decisions I had to confront. I was resentful of mother's illness, which I didn't even want to know more about. I wanted to avoid it and, unfortunately, the medical caregivers allowed me to do just that. What a mistake.

Her doctor was kind, but of limited help. I accompanied Mother on visits to his office, and that is just what they were—visits. He would chatter about her medications and her heart, concerning himself with blood pressure, pulse, and other general "busy-makers." I would ask about her change of moods at night. Why was she wandering around the house unable to sleep, stuffing things in plastic bags and calling the neighbors at three in the morning? He would smile and prescribe a sleeping pill. When that didn't work, he gave her a larger dosage. We would bid the doctor goodbye and return home to face the terrors that began to grow heavier and heavier. In his chatty way the doctor once opined that Mother had "a little senile dementia," adding, "but most people her age do." She was seventy-seven at the time, and as both she and the disease grew older, our knowledge, our patience, and our understanding did not improve.

Mom was still driving then, and when she shut the car door on her leg, forgetting to pull it in before slamming the door shut, we chalked it up to one of the silly things old people do. But it worried us, she had hurt herself badly. When she couldn't remember how to write checks we did it for her, and she signed them. More "old age." When she got lost at church and couldn't find her way home, we began to think, "That's old age?" We were concerned but, after all, "it only happened once." I have heard caregivers say this a thousand times. *It only happened once.* I have since learned that if it happens once, it will probably happen again and maybe again. Actually, such excuses allowed us to avoid tough decisions such as taking the car away from her. We needed help, but did not know it, and we accepted what was happening to her, never, never opening our eyes to what was coming. She would forget, I would yell, and time passed.

We joked that she couldn't smell any longer. We'd say, "Don't give Grandma any perfumes for Christmas because she surely can't smell them." We'd walk through perfume departments at the stores and laugh that she didn't smell a thing in that cacophony of odors. We did not know that this is true of many Alzheimer's patients if the disease happens to attack that part of the brain.

We thought that perhaps her hearing might be causing some of her problems. One thousand dollars later, we went to get "the device" installed. This would solve everything. We just knew that she asked the same question over because she hadn't heard the answer. Sorry. It didn't help. But the thousand dollars did buy one thing. In four sessions at the hearing center I discovered the sad truth that no learning was going on. I may not have understood Alzheimer's, but as a teacher, I understood learning and Mother *could not learn.* Usually by dent of enough repetitions, a person can be taught to do a simple task, but the circuits were obviously dead or dying in Mother's brain. I had to face it. She could *not* learn to put that thing into her ear, and she had absolutely no idea of how to adjust the volume. That was that. A dead ear and a brain no longer functional for learning. Alarm bell number two went off in my brain. I didn't care what the doctor said. This had to be more than old age.

It was noon and the medicine jar was empty:

> "Mother, where is your evening medicine?"
> "I don't know. Isn't it there?"
> "Mother, when did you take your medicine?"
> "Oh, I don't think I took them at all. I'm sorry!"

This began to be a daily pattern and, angry and frightened, I had to figure another more foolproof way of regulating her medicines. I hid them and gave them to her as she needed them with her standing there telling me I was poisoning her.

As time went on, Mother's dark moods became even darker and her suspicions of anyone around her grew apace. She hallucinated about naked little boys in her living room. She was convinced the furniture in her apartment "only looked like the real thing." She was sure someone had stolen the real furniture. Several times she called the neighbors in the middle of the night asking them to come get her at the railroad station. They would sleepily call and alert us that "Mother's downstairs

looking for home." Our nights during this period were short and inter-
rupted. Mother would roam the house until about three A.M. and then
pass out somewhere until seven. The medication which the doctor pre-
scribed did little good, yet that was all he could offer.

When alarm bell number three sounded, I was totally unprepared. I
can remember it so clearly, even though it happened years ago. I stood
in the kitchen getting breakfast, the coffeepot bubbling away on the
counter. Mother came up the stairs from her apartment wrapped in a
beautiful Pennsylvania quilt with blood running down her face and over
the quilt. My husband and I ran to her and started trying to make sense
of this trauma patient before us. The blood, luckily, was caked and
dried, and there was no fresh bleeding. The damage seemed to be a very
large, ugly cut over her right eye.

She had no idea what had happened to her. Looking back, I don't
think she even realized she was hurt. Our panic frightened her, and our
questioning seemed to awaken her to the fact that something was seriously wrong. Quickly, we bundled her into a coat and took her to the
emergency room. I had found her broken glasses in her bedroom near
the dresser. Apparently she had bumped her head on the dresser and
broken the glasses, which had then caused the cut. Many stitches later,
she still didn't remember what had happened. She was a total blank
slate. Had she immediately realized she had fallen and alerted us, that
would have been understandable. But apparently, she had simply folded
the quilt around her and had gone peacefully to sleep, totally unaware
that she was injured and bleeding. Had the cut been deeper, she could
have bled to death.

This time the alarm was clanging loudly in my head. Unless we could
watch her twenty-four hours a day, Mother was no longer safe alone.
What if she fell while we were sleeping or at work and did nothing? At
this point in every Alzheimer's case, a decision must be made to either
prevent a crisis and see that she is safe or to let the crisis happen. I would
never try to make that decision for any other family but, *at that time,* I
couldn't let a crisis happen, no matter what. That was the bell that woke
me up to what we were fighting. Senility, my foot! Give her a sleeping
pill, my eye! I didn't know what was happening to Mother, but I was beginning to see that it had a very evil side.

Shortly after this, I called her personal doctor, told him what had happened, and asked for an explanation. How could this be a simple case of senility? It was then July, and I would have to begin teaching in the fall. I could see that Mother wasn't safe alone in the daytime and, under direct questioning, the doctor said she probably needed twenty-four hour around-the-clock care.

I asked for a complete battery of tests to determine what was causing her illness. Surely we could discover something treatable and return her to her previous health. For some reason the doctor placed Mother in the hospital for these tests, probably thinking this would be the easiest way to get the job done. What a mistake that was. At that time hospitals were not good at dealing with dementia. I'm not sure they are that much better today, but most doctors now usually run tests on an out-patient basis knowing the wreckage that a hospital visit can cause a demented person.

But that was then, and they took Mother at face value. She looked small and inoffensive, sweet and demure, and they accepted her as such. Big mistake. Like a small but wicked child, Mother was soon racing up and down the halls, chatting with everyone, entering the men's room at will, and generally being the biggest pest in the world. They quickly shuffled her to the medical floor and had a nurse's aide keep a close watch on her. Unfortunately, Mother didn't like having her wings clipped, and she promptly began throwing coffee cups at nurses, aides, or anyone who tried to suppress her.

The staff was finally forced to restrain her to keep from having to sedate her while they tested. The difficulty of testing an Alzheimer's patient became obvious when they tried to get a urine sample. They had to hold her down and give her a catheter. Later, all of the nurses were shaking their heads and muttering about Mother's hysterical screams during *that* maneuver. They couldn't understand why she had become so upset. Couldn't understand? Later Mother told me that they had raped her, and she was sure it happened on the floor of the grocery store in her old hometown—a small example of how Alzheimer's destroys communication.

The conclusion of this horrendous three weeks (I have never understood why it took three weeks) was that nothing showed in the blood work or the X-rays, given then instead of CAT scans or an MRI. All we knew was that she showed significant loss of cognitive function. The resulting diagnosis was probable Alzheimer's.

I remember the day my husband and I sat in the family room at the hospital. Ann, a registered nurse well versed in Alzheimer's, explained to us, "Your mother has lost a significant part of her short-term memory and is rapidly losing her ability to do most things for herself. She should not be left alone." She described a nursing home to us where, in the Alzheimer's wing, patients are gradually weaned from drug dependency and given freedom to wander and roam at will.

At her suggestion we visited this facility. On the surface it was much like any well-appointed nursing home, but there was a feeling about it that intrigued me. Nurses, aides, and patients were all chattering together and it was often difficult to decide who were the patients. Those patients, so disposed, wandered at will, inside and out, protected from leaving the site by a high wooden fence. One group sat in the center of the room tossing balloons to one another. In a corner an aide was going through an animal picture book, encouraging a patient to name each creature. Debbie, another patient, was playing away at the piano and a few ladies were warbling accompaniment. A cat wandered around the edges of the activity, haughtily ignoring much of what was going on but finally finding a friendly lap to inhabit.

Fortunately, I had been led to one of the most progressive Alzheimer's units in the Denver area. Directed by Ann Collings, whose mother died of Alzheimer's, the patients there were truly loved and attended to. I realized that I could not offer my mother what these professionals were able to give. I would be gone all day teaching and she would either be dangerously alone or housebound with an in-house aide. Adult day centers were, at this time, minimally present. I asked Ann what they would do if Mother wandered at night; would they give sleeping pills? She answered, "We will let her wander." Under Ann's expert guidance, almost all medicines, except Mother's heart medicines, were discarded (this was before the days of Aricept, Excelon, and others), and Mother's sundowning began to subside.

Those who have gone this way before know what happened next. As Alice said in *Wonderland,* "It got curiouser and curiouser." Skipping ahead three years, we look in on her at the home. There she sits. She wears slacks I've never seen, a baggy, ragged sweater she refuses to change, and two different house slippers. Her nose runs, but she doesn't remember to wipe it with one of the eternally present tissues in her pocket. She has on someone else's glasses, and she has long ago flushed her dentures down the toilet. I remember this time so well. It was the day that Mother taught me that life is short and we need to seize every day.

> She asked me, "Where is my daddy?"
> I answered, "He died when you were three years old, Mom."
> "Oh, my! How old am I now?" she wanted to know.
> "You're eighty-five," I answered. A startled look came over her
> face and she focused intensely on my eyes and said,
> "I am? Eighty-five? Where did she go?"

Where indeed? Her pronouns were definitely garbled and her sentences confused, but by this time I had learned to listen to her underlying messages. This message came through loud and clear, and I thought my heart was breaking. Where had she gone, indeed. The poor soul thought she was a young child and this person sitting beside her had told her she was eighty-five. I had stolen her entire life without knowing it.

On some visits she abandoned the poor little girl personality and became a bit more arrogant, continually shaking her leg as though her motor was running but no one was at the controls. The machinery was on idle and obviously not functioning. But there she was. She was my mother, yet in my mind she was no mother of mine. I wished I could get her a permanent, but she would have screamed so loudly the beautician wouldn't have touched her. I wished I could have fixed her up pretty. She had been so beautiful. No, I couldn't do that. The clothes disappeared, the makeup was eaten, mirrors got broken, and she lost her false teeth. I wondered if she would like a new pair of slippers. That was something I could do. A week later she was wearing two different slippers. She had hidden the mates. This dreadful disease thwarted all our good intentions, even the least of them.

As a stranger took the place of the mother of my youth, I did not realize how desperately I would miss her. There she sat, my mother, but in my heart I had had her funeral. The mother of my childhood memories was no longer present. I wanted so much to tell her about her new great-grandson.

"Mom, do you remember Jon?"

"What? Well, well. Can you stay? The work is hard here."

"Well, Mom, Jon just had a boy baby, and they named him Clinton, just like Dad."

"Clinton. I've heard of him. Is he your son? They take everything here. See her? She's mean to me."

"Mom, did you hear what I said?"

"Said, sad? Oh, yes I'm sooooooo sad."

My *one of a kind* mother was irrevocably lost. Blessedly, we did have our moments during the long siege. All was not sadness and pain.

There she sat with legs outstretched before her as her brain progressively refused to send the body any message to bend. She looked through me as though I wasn't there. Charles walked by putting salt and pepper shakers in his pants. The aides were looking for Frank's trousers. What's that in Mom's arms? It's Frank's trousers. How did she get them? We didn't ask.

Many days were too sad to remember until much later, a tiny bit at a time. The day I tried to give her a kiss and she stiffened and asked, "Who are you?" No kisses on that day. She was not about to kiss a stranger and that is what I was to her on that day. I was not in that day's dream. I was not wanted and she suggested I leave. My mother with the open arms was lost, gone forever. I drove home, trying to avoid the traffic through my tears.

Finally, about eight years after it began, at the age of eighty-six, she lay in her final coma, the smell of death all about her. Mother had not signed a living will, and the hardest decisions of my life were upon me. Should I put her on an I.V.? She had an infection. Should we give her an antibiotic? Death had come to claim what little was left of her frail frame and we did nothing to prevent it. It hovered over her, paused for a while, and quietly took her breath. Gently, she went very gently. My irreplaceable mother was gone for the last time. The end, the end, the end.

And yet, there she sits in my mind's eye. "Please don't leave me as a fragmented memory. Please make some sense of all this pain." And so I've picked up the pieces, returned to the house that is now in ashes, and asked myself how I could have helped her more. Was there any meaning in her final illness? Why had she had to suffer in such a terrible way?

I couldn't begin to answer these questions in the immediate years after Mother's death. According to an article by Marge Dempsey and Sylvia Braago, professionals associated with the Alzheimer's Society of the Niagara Region in Ontario, the loss upon the illness and final death of an Alzheimer's loved one is greater than we realize at the time. In their research on latent grief they identify three dimensions of loss for the caregiver.

First, there is the *loss of the person*—the mother, sister, friend, and partner—and the roles he or she has played in our lives. I had gradually lost my mother in the swing, my best friend, and my grandchildren's great-grandmother. Second, there is the *symbolic loss* of the dreams and expectations that we nurture for years. Retirement dreams are all erased. In my mother's case, eight years of happy times were lost to oblivion and dementia. Third is the *caregiver's loss of self* or personal identity. We are required to assume new roles formerly held by the loved one. This happens so suddenly that we are unable to adjust. I had to become my mother's mother. She had become a three-year-old child. Our relationship, as it had been, no longer existed and, in a way, part of me had disappeared. I no longer was a daughter. I no longer was a part of this "something" that we had together.

And as Dempsey and Braago state, "The loved one is irretrievably lost, but the caregiver, in his fragmented state, must find himself and become whole again in order to live on" (84–91).

During her illness, I never cried. I was ashen inside. The vital spark of my life was damaged much more from within than from without. No external influence can hurt us as much as the damage we do ourselves. I was devastated by my loss and hers. My mother was a family "chaser." She had haunted county archives, rubbed tombstones, and made millions of scrawly notes concerning her family history, proudly displaying her Daughters of the Revolution certificate. She collected old pictures, letters tied with ribbons, notes on scraps of paper, baskets, china, and other treasures from her family history. Alzheimer's took all this away from her. The lady who loved her family and her history could remember neither. She lived her last years thinking she was totally alone.

The day she lost her family was the day I lost my God. I could tell that it was not a good day when I approached her. Alzheimer's patients have good days and bad, and this one was going to be particularly tricky. Tears were streaming down her small face, and her hands plucked at my sleeve. "Who are you?" she asked. I swallowed the pain that this lack of recognition brought and answered:

> "Why, Mom, I'm your daughter."
> "Oh, good!" She was elated and the tears stopped momentarily. "I thought I didn't have any family. I thought I was all alone and nobody loved me." She clutched my arm so tightly I was afraid to move.
> "So, what is your name?" she asked in all seriousness.

For the moment, the tears stopped, but they would come again. She would soon forget what I had told her and the loneliness and fear would return to haunt her, all alone with no past and no future. And in Alzheimer's this happens over and over and over again.

I didn't actually lose my God that day. I just misplaced him. My father's cancer hadn't affected my assurances. Death at age seventy-nine is sad, traumatic, and full of grief, yet it is to be expected. Although I had been very close to my father, I felt no sense of disorder in the universe because of his death. It was as it had to be. However, when Mother became ill with Alzheimer's, anger welled up inside me at the unfairness of it all. How dare God give my sweet mom this dreadful disease! How dare He take her family and memories away from her! How dare He strip her of her dignity! How dare He! But He did.

My prayers went unanswered, and Mother had deteriorated into a disoriented, mumbling caricature. Her French-rolled hairdo became a tangled mess, and I was left seething at a God who obviously didn't love Mother or He would not have visited her with such a crushing burden. "God is good, God is love, and God is The Father." A good and loving Father would not, I repeat, would not, could not, do this to my innocent, gentle mother.

I began to realize that a lot of my pain was due to my own attitude. Yes, I had an *attitude*. I didn't think anyone could help me help Mother. I turned a blind eye to friends, colleagues, and professionals, preferring to listen to my own tune. Unfortunately, I had no tune. I had never walked this path before. I needed guidance and kind friends, but I was blocking myself off from such help.

It was long after Mother's death that I began to mend. Deep grief caused me to begin to tend my own garden, going back and searching for meaning in what had passed. Before I realized it, overlooked buds of knowledge and faith began to emerge, softening the hardened anguish. I could once again cry. In my newfound maturity I picked fruit from any tree that offered substance. I turned to poetry and the classics and found much there. I loved Henry David Thoreau's musings after the death of his brother.

> *Only nature has a right to grieve perpetually,*
> *for she only is innocent. Soon the ice will melt,*
> *and the blackbirds sing along the river,*
> *which he frequented, as pleasantly as ever.*
> *The same everlasting serenity will appear*
> *in this face of God, and we will*
> *not be sorrowful, if he is not.*
> —Henry David Thoreau, *The Journals*

I am an unconsecrated gardener. In spring I love the new buds, the encroaching greens, and the idea of planting beauteous garden patches. But many things about gardening are not all sunshine and golden beauty. Spading and turning over soil is difficult, and hoeing a patch of claylike loam is not very pleasant. Like life, the garden has its beauty and its thorns. Certain plants, if I'm not careful, may kill my dogs. Some days I come in scratched and dirty from time among the growing rose bushes. Yet I know the arduous days are somehow necessary to allow a beautiful outcome. Without the difficult days and dirty work, I might not see the beauty before my eyes.

And then there was Job. I read the book over several times and found that at the end the answer is, "I AM," saith the Lord. God rained trials and pestilences on Job, and in the end there was nothing but God saying, "Regardless of what else, I AM." In my own mind I accepted this

to mean, "This is the way it is. The trials and pain are part of the blessing of life." I believe it was Queen Elizabeth who said, at the memorial
for British subjects who died in the World Towers tragedy, "Grief is the
price we pay for love." What a beautiful sentiment.

I began to see Mother's suffering and the suffering of us all as a natural part of the life's pain, the sacrifice we give for the joy of living. I will
not cry. The blackbirds are singing.

THREE
The Most Hurtful Things

All pain is not created equal. Some things hurt worse than others. As Roseanne Roseanna Danna, Gilda Radner's famous character, liked to say, "It's always something," and with Alzheimer's, this is true. It is also true that some of its most vicious thrusts cut with a pain like nothing ever hurt before. To me, watching the personality of the person I loved disappear killed me, and when she no longer knew who I was it broke my heart. The fact that she asked incessantly to "go home," while I was powerless to grant her wish tore me apart. These are special hurts to the Alzheimer's family and they deserve a chapter of their own.

Where Is My Person?

A caregiver said to me recently, "I hate this THING that I have to take care of." In tears, she continued, "My dear, sweet, loving mother is gone. I want her back. NOW!" Alzheimer's is an impatient thief. It kills before it allows death to happen and it maims the most vulnerable part of the body—the brain. As it destroys each tiny neuron, we lose our loved ones, inch by inch, cell by cell. Often, outsiders are unaware of what is happening because it happens so slowly, but we see it. We see the destruction coming, we see the disease strike over and over, and we lose our person again and again. We stand by, unable to do anything, watching. Each morning when we wake to see our person, we hold our breaths. What part has been chipped away today? Will it be her sweet smile, the way he puts his arm around me, or the feeling of camaraderie we have when we share a private moment?

At first, when I looked at Mother, it was still Mother. Like the picture within the picture, what I saw was the shell, the frame. The externals were all still there but with each glance the personality grows smaller and smaller until at last, when I looked into her eyes, all I saw was a vacancy. She was escaping me only to be replaced by a frightened little girl or an angry, imperious, demanding queen, depending on the mood of the moment. With most illnesses, the mind is there until the end. You don't lose the personhood of the one you love until you also lose the body. Alzheimer's introduces you to a stranger, or in some instances, to several strange personalities. Getting used to them is half the battle. To love them is the other half of the battle.

Somehow, some way, the family wrestles through these years, desperately trying to do what is best and watching the slow unwinding of their loved one. Sad to say, many caregivers are left feeling that they have bungled the job. Where did Mother go? What happened to her? What did I do wrong? As one caregiver told me, "I just don't know where to go to get help." It is mind-boggling.

I would venture to say that in ninety percent of the cases, we didn't do anything wrong. It is just the face of Alzheimer's playing hide-and-seek. Looking back, I wish that I had been more diligent in searching for the mother I was losing. Had I watched carefully, I might have gotten a bigger peek at the emotional side of her. God bless her soul. After all, she never stopped enjoying a hug and a kiss, an observation that recent research has vindicated. One approach to reaching the Alzheimer's patient is by a gentle appeal to his or her emotions. One caregiver recently told me that she couldn't get her mother to take her medications until she started to joke with her and say, "Okay, come on now, let's all take our happy pills." Something about this light-hearted approach did the trick and the task was accomplished.

The problem is, however, that for most of us the abusive remarks, anger, and fear are taken too personally and keep us from offering intelligent solutions to emotional behavior. We don't know this new person that is being created by the disease, and we have to brace ourselves to offer affection, steeling ourselves for the paranoid response, the angry words, the personal insults or, what can be worse, a total lack of understanding. We try, and sometimes we can communicate with our mother, our *old* mother, but at other times we are just not in her present dream and have to accept the rebuff. So, what is left for us?

Can the reader imagine the depression that the gradual loss of a loved one can cause? It breaks the heart. Bill and Lois are in their retirement years, and Bill had been looking forward to time for the two of them to share intellectual interests and travel dreams. Bill is a retired minister and, being a man of thoughtful mien, he suffers with her in this transition from person to personality. In answer to a letter inquiring about his health, he writes:

> How are things with me right now? Lousy! Lois has been deteriorating in the last few weeks at a pace I can hardly believe. She has no energy, no appetite, and "doesn't feel well" constantly. A part of the latter is that she is recovering from a bout with the flu and had a cyst removed from her lip a week and a half ago and "it still hurts." She doesn't change out of her gown and robe unless the kids are coming down to visit. Her only occupation is to sit on the living room couch and work on her puzzle book. Our daughter talked her into a much shorter hairstyle about three weeks ago and she hates it. Consequently, she refuses to go back to the beauty shop and doesn't have the energy to do it herself.
>
> All of this brings ME to a new point. Caregivers comment on how the person they have known isn't there any longer. Well, I'm finally beginning to know the depths of that. I thought I did before, but I didn't. At times I feel like I'm living with a zombie. I don't mean to be a crybaby, but right now that's what I feel like doing. The only trouble is, I can't cry because it would further upset this woman whom I still love.

Rather than let Lois see his pain, Bill let his grief build up inside of him to the point where his own health was in danger. In protecting her, he was in danger of destroying himself. This is the most unexpected—and one of the most sinister—results of Alzheimer's. We grieve for each loss, as at a death, but we have no accepted public receptacle for that grief. We hesitate to let our loved one see our sorrow. There are no funerals for the living dead. Wounded, we cry in private and mourn a death that is yet to be, and yet is happening before us twenty-four hours a day, day after day.

Grieving Our Own Loss

As the relationship changes, as the person changes, so do we. When we grieve, we mourn the loss, not only of our loved one, but also the loss of our relationship with that person. The rapport we had with our loved one before Alzheimer's struck is destroyed. We miss the camaraderie and the sharing of stories. We crave the affection and caresses that we were

wont to receive. Our loved one keeps asking to "go home" and, ironically, that is what we want to do, too. With Alzheimer's, both the caregiver and the patient need comforting.

David lives in Adelaide, South Australia and is the single caregiver for
his Alzheimer's "Mum." Since 1998, David has been her around-the-
clock caregiver. "She has gone from being fiercely independent to totally
dependent," he says. He recaptures a moment of ever-waning closeness
when he shares this glimpse of his mother:

> Just peeked into the lounge. Mum was very asleep in her chair
> after a trip to the doctor today. On the floor just in front of her was
> the cat, also very asleep. I got that warm gooey feeling inside. You
> know the one. You get it when you've just arrived home after a big
> day out with the kids, a long drive home, and there they are fast
> asleep in the back, not a worry in the world. Sometimes I get that
> feeling at night when I look in on her in bed and the cat is curled up
> next to her. It may not be the dictionary version, but a family still
> does live in this house, and this house is a home. I think it's nap-
> time.

To David, his mother has always been family, home, love, and comfort.
This momentary glimpse of her reassures him that he has not yet lost it
all. The two of them are still "family." We grasp, we cling, and we fight
for this continuity of warmth.

The parents of J. were coming for a Christmas visit. She had been
Daddy's little girl and had started to sense the change in their relationship. How could she interact with him if she was no longer his little girl?
Were there any grounds for companionship? Add to this the fact that
she hadn't seen him for some time, and she knew the change would
shock her. This letter reflects her conflicted emotions:

> I feel so stupid. I'm forty-eight but feel like a little kid that is un-
> able to learn her ABC's. Dad is coming to visit and I guess you could
> say I feel really nervous being around him. I know this sounds hor-
> rid, but I just sort of try to ignore him when he visits. I really feel
> he's dead to me. He and I used to be the closest buddies. I could
> confide anything to my father. Now that he's lost the old days, I just
> can't talk to him anymore. I know I should be more loving toward
> him but just can't do it.

Looking back, I know that we have to be gentle with ourselves for feeling alienated. To watch this slow unraveling of someone we love and respect is beyond endurance. We all want to do what I did today in a particularly violent movie. I stuck my fingers in my ears and closed my eyes, anything to protect the senses.

Now that Mother is gone, I am beginning to piece together a sense of human connectedness that differs from the one I had pre-Alzheimer's. I think sociologists are right when they say that we are made up of the many roles we play in life. However, I sense that beyond our roles lies a ME who is always there. J.'s father is unable to act out his "role" as father, but he is still there. He can still be reached. Perhaps if we learn a different language and choose a different look, we may be able to gain precious new information about the real daddy. Alzheimer's often makes us realize that we are myopic and demand to see our loved one in a role he or she has held that makes *us* feel comfortable.

Amazingly, when the verbal avenues are blocked, the spirit often finds a tactile, sensory, or even a spiritual sixth sense to guide it. The heart learns new ways to communicate, and we can intuitively sense subtleties about our loved one that we had not known previously. When this happens, we suddenly realize that, in some strange way, Alzheimer's has deepened our lives and loves. These are often the memories we cherish once our loved one has gone forever. The emotional connections between us can become deeper than they ever were before.

If I could have given any advice to J., it would have been to let the spirit of the season take over. Hold your father's hand, look into his eyes. Smile and let him know that it's all right, that we'll take care of everything. Tell him you love him.

I dream of having Mother back for just one more Christmas moment, to sit beside her and let the silence talk. I dream that I would keep the season simple for her, as simple and peaceful and as lacking in distractions as possible. I so wish she were still here, so that I could practice my own "wise words." I deeply miss that little Alzheimer's person who was present after the mother role was spent. Looking back, I wish I had missed the mother less and loved the Alzheimer's person more. That's where many good memories are.

Dreams do not simply show us what we know.
They tell us more than we know; they remind us
there are many ways of knowing.
—Nancy Willard, *Telling Time*

Easily said. However, it is not always possible in the middle of some Alzheimer's stages to maintain a lofty outlook. Our need for rational control over our lives can prevent us from any loving communication with a demented loved one. Gloria has had to relocate her mother and deal with some very violent behavior. She confesses:

> I frequently find myself looking at my loved one and wondering who really is inside of her. There are times that I simply do not recognize this person I am caring for, and she is in a relatively early stage. Throughout my life, she was always my staunchest supporter and closest friend. Now, when she is accusing me and screaming at me like a shrew, I find my inner dialogue telling me that I hate her, that I hate my situation, and that I hate my loss of freedom; I hate hearing her stories over and over again, and I hate the sound of her voice.
>
> Then I spend the rest of the day in the deepest, darkest pit of guilt one can imagine. The scariest thing is that I am getting to the point where I can barely recognize myself. It is a strange experience to look into the mirror and wonder who is looking back at you.
>
> The idea of writing down our blackest thoughts is a good idea because it acts as a catharsis for those of us who have never been able to verbalize for fear of a giant thunderbolt coming out of the blue to strike us. Speaking of dark thoughts, there are days when I would welcome that thunderbolt.

Every time this anger surfaces it creates one more destructive memory to face when we make that inevitable return journey. Hate my mother? How could I feel that way? We have to remember that we are not perfect.

Becoming A Stranger

The day comes when our loved one doesn't know us. This is close to unbearable. Our person has been chiseled away until there is no relationship between us. Until that sad day we can deny that there is substantial change, but on that day of non-recognition, we feel as unimportant to our loved one as any stranger. Some children and grandchildren cannot bear to visit after this happens. Spouses feel desolate and as though their efforts to nurture are totally useless. *Why should I go visit her? She doesn't even know who I am.* Stubbornly, we refuse to take the new creature into our hearts. "That's not Grandma!"

Jerry, a long-time caregiver, comforts someone new to the disease:

> In regard to your mother not knowing who you are, I'm glad it was only for a day. I go through this every day now with Mother. Earlier this week she was having a fit about going home and was mad at me for keeping her in this prison and not letting her go to see her children. I sat down in front of her and asked her to look at me. When she did, I asked her who I was. She looked at me really hard and then said, "I have no idea who you are. I've never seen you before in my life. Why are you keeping me locked up here?"
>
> And there's no point in denying it. It hurts to know that I'm now a perfect stranger to my mother, even though I've seen it coming. Now whenever my wife, my mother, and I go out anywhere together, Mom will tell my wife, "Please don't you go off and leave me alone with this man." Of course, all my wife and I can do is laugh about it. There's no point in trying to reassure her anymore as she's unable to grasp the reality of what we're telling her.

What a wrenching, provoking emotion to have quit one's job, as Jerry did, in order to care for his Mom and then she says, "Don't leave me alone with this man." One would not blame him much if he walked out and left the scene. But the caregiver realizes this is not a rational scene. This is not the time to take such a step. It is a time to count to ten, to take the moment for what it is, just a moment. It will pass. But inwardly, in our more secret, soft places, the hurt grows larger.

Lori has faced her mother's confusion on occasion, but she explains when it will hurt the very worst:

> There seem to be more and more occasions when my Alzheimer's mom doesn't know me. She has been living with us for five years, since about the time she was diagnosed, and has been in stage six for a long time. The decline has been very gradual over the last four years. This is the first change I've noticed in a while and it's still only part of the time.

My sister and I always find it interesting that when we talk to people about our Alzheimer's mother, the first question they always ask is, "Does she still know you?" Whether Mom knows me has never been that important to me, even when she failed to recognize me the first time over four years ago. I always felt it was more important that Mom was happy, comfortable, and healthy.

But, now that there are more occasions that Mom is confused about who I am, I've realized the down side. Tonight when I was telling her how much I love her, she smiled politely and said, "How could that be? You hardly know me!"

I much prefer it when Mom first sees me in the morning and her face lights up. She smiles so wide and says, "There's my little girl!" We hug and hug. When her weekday caregiver brings her home from an outing and I greet Mom coming in, she says, "Here she is! Come here, Honey!"

I say, "I love when you call me 'Honey.'"

And she says, "Well, Honey, I just love you so much. And I missed you." Even when I goof up a recipe and feign discouragement I can count on her to tell me, "That's all right, Honey. It looks good! No one will know the difference," while she hugs me and strokes my hair back, that little forehead massage that moms do.

It's not just that I love being loved. It's also that Mom is most herself when it comes to loving. She's lost so much to this disease, so many capabilities and so much of her personality, but she has never forgotten how to give and receive love. She can't form a complete sentence with real words that make sense or isn't made up unless, it seems, she's communicating love. When she's loving me, I can forget that she has Alzheimer's disease.

I imagine as my mom knows me less and less she will still appreciate me. But it means I'm losing the one part of her that hadn't changed: the loving mother. If she does not recognize me as her daughter, she cannot love me like my mother any more. And I will never be able to pretend she's Alzheimer's-free again, which will be a turning point in caregiving for me. We don't have too many people in this world who love us *unconditionally* and to lose a significant one is a huge loss; but to lose them before they're really gone hurts terribly and, with Alzheimer's, it hurts over and over.

Lori expresses so well what we caregivers call the Long Goodbye or, more aptly, the Living Death. She has lost the unconditional love of her mother years before her mother has physically departed.

Sometimes we can wisely avoid the recognition trap. This caregiver shows us that attitude is all:

> And so I stopped asking if she knew who I was. I would wait to see how Mother saw me and try to react to that. Her big smile of recognition became enough, and if I got a hug—wow! I could live for a week. What more could I ask for? Recognition? Yes, I needed a sign that I had not lost my identity in her eyes. But Alzheimer's denied me that. Sometimes she thought I was her mother, and I tried to be satisfied with that, remembering that my grandmother was a strong, kind woman, and it was really a compliment to be compared to her.
>
> But I had to remind myself that these are the days of giving love, not receiving it. Goodbye to love unconditional, hello to payback days. These were the days when I must try to give back all she's given me and, in many cases, I may have to give back more. It's so easy to be loved and so comforting, so seemingly arid to give without the recompense of recognition. Perhaps these are the days that test our valor and character, the days when we earn our stripes. To give without return is the highest form of giving. Isn't it?
>
> I didn't know just how difficult it was going to be to view her as a feeling, willful, mortal being as the disease progressed. Now I had to tend to the care of someone I didn't know anymore. I had to accept that this person came into my mother's body and took charge. There is no more profoundly difficult task that a caregiver shoulders than to care for the unloved. Or to learn to love the Alzheimer's stranger.

One of the strange things about Alzheimer's that neither caregiver mentions is something called *Capgras Syndrome*. This is the stage in the disease when the patient recognizes you both as you are and as you were. Your loved one may ask where you are and argue that you may be who you are but not who he or she is looking for. The patient may talk about two different versions of the same you, like the person facing them and "that other one." It's a common symptom of the disease, but if you try to be rational about it, it can lead to frustration on everyone's part. Just put on the double yoke of recognition and be happy for the duplication.

Mary Lou lives in Minnesota and has been in charge of her mother's care for nearly four years. Before that she was involved long distance in her mother's care for about two years:

It's been a year or so since Mom really knew who I was. It seemed to happen gradually. Now, more often than not, she'll ask my name. I'll tell her it's Mary Lou. Then she tells me I don't look like her. In an odd moment she once said she thought Mary Lou was about ten years old, maybe a little younger.

For a long time she would tell me all about Mary Lou. She was Mom's pal who did lots of things with her—shop, go out to eat, go for rides, play games, etc.—someone she had a good time with. "We were good pals, but suddenly she stopped visiting," Mom said. We were still doing all those things, but to her I was someone else, not the Mary Lou she remembered. Hearing her say her pal had quit visiting hurt worse than the idea that she didn't know who I was.

Now when I visit, she often tells me that my being there does her no good and I might as well leave. Sometimes I stay and sometimes I go. Either way, it is painful to be unable to help. Once again she wants to go home and virtually no diversions will sway her from that goal. She says she's hungry, but when food is offered she'll eat only a bite or two and then quit, saying she can't eat any more because she wants to go home.

Where Oh Where Is Home?

One seriously painful part of Alzheimer's is the loved one's search for home that Mary Lou mentions. Alzheimer's is a demented world teeming with the homeless, people who want to go somewhere if only they could figure out where. It is an obvious cry for help that we cannot answer. We want to cry out, "If you just tell us where home is, we'll try to take you there." A few years ago I wrote about this painful aspect of Alzheimer's:

> Her frazzled white hair in disarray, she stands by the nursing home door asking to go home. Her birdlike hands twist around her handbag, and her tiny face looks too small for the sweatsuit outfit she wears. She peers out of her favorite red colored turtleneck top, searching, always searching for something that is secure, something that makes sense. "Please, please, won't someone take me home?" Her purse hangs over her arm, banging into the door and entering guests as she pushes up against them.

At some point in this disease, almost all Alzheimer's patients want to "go home." The puzzle for the family is, "Where is home?" If our loved one is in a nursing home, guilt keeps us awake at night and we have nightmares about the separation anxiety our dear one must be feeling. I have heard aides gossip about how families "dump" relatives and then never visit. "*That* must be why they want to go home so bad," they whisper.

If you have ever seen the little lady I described above, you too will want to rap someone for neglect. Even though the sad truth is that many old persons *are* neglected, in the majority of cases the Alzheimer's victim may be "at home" and still want to "go home." Mother lived in an apartment downstairs from us for years before we had to put her in a special-care unit. Supposedly she knew we were upstairs asleep, but about once or twice a week she would panic and want to "go home." "No this furniture isn't mine," she would argue. "Mine is at home!" Home may have been the childhood home where Mom and Dad ruled and provided the security she now seeks. Maybe it is just a refuge, a symbol for comfort and safety, or a need for love.

Jerry Ham lives in Washington state and first became aware of his mother's problem following her breast surgery in 1991. Jerry grieves because his mother's illness seems to have contributed to the heart problem that took his father in 1995. Trying desperately to care for his wife, Jerry's father put off the heart surgery too long. Since his father's death, Jerry has cared for his mother in his home. Jerry describes his mother's quest for home:

> Mother has lived with us for over a year now, and she still wants to go home, but when asked where home is, she can't remember. She lived in Edmonds, Washington for nearly twenty-eight years before we moved her here to our home. For the next few months, she would threaten to kill me, if necessary, in order to get back home.
>
> Even now, Mother often stands at the window and looks out muttering, "I've got to go home." When I ask why, she replies that her children need her and don't know where to find her. Or, "I've got to go home to check on Mother because she needs me and will be worried about me if I don't get home." Her mother passed away in 1974. Yesterday she was in her room and very upset. When I inquired why, she said, "Daddy's going to be really worried about me if I don't get home." She gets quite emotional about it, and yet I

know that if we were to just drive by her former home in Edmonds, she would not be able to recognize it.

Some of the darkest days of my life were in the middle of Mother's illness when I would visit her, and her little hands would hold me ever so tight, tight enough to hurt, and she would ask me to take her home. "Why can't I live with you?" she would plead, her smile coyly trying to convince, her eyes asking for a sign of agreement, her hand plucking at my sleeve. Her pleas caused me to search and pray about ways to keep her at home. Two years after her death I still had dreams in which she got so much better that we decided to bring her home. But, in fact, God had to do that. God had to take her home.

Home is love, home is security, and home is the solution to all problems. That's why we flinch when we hear our loved one ask to "go home." Try as we will, we will never be able to make them feel secure ever again. The anxiety and the demands of this disease forever holds them in a frightening world of total uncertainty: no memories, no future, no hope.

We have to accept the pain that comes as Mother turns to say goodbye to the home she has loved and now must leave. We have to ache when a spouse doesn't feel safe living with his loved one. "You mean my husband no longer feels that home is with me?" Our loved ones move on to another dimension, and we can only grasp a hand, hug a shoulder, or caress a cheek and whisper, "Love is home, and I love you," until they fade completely away.

Gradually, we learn to cope. We begin to take one day at a time, and we try not to overreact to behaviors that once reduced us to tears. We begin to realize that their recognition of us is not as important as our recognition of their needs. By providing them with more security, we find ways to help them find home.

In hindsight, I realize that these years were an important part of Mother's life. To be embarrassed by her or to be annoyed because she didn't know me was beside the point. What was really happening was that I was being given an opportunity. I was being given an opportunity to learn to love a person I had not met before. I raged at losing my mother, but now I see how wonderful this uninhibited little Alzheimer's mom was.

My Own Little Bum

Toward the end of her illness, my Alzheimer's Mom was, at times, a frightened mite of a thing, sometimes wanting nothing more than to cuddle in my arms, a wounded bird seeking shelter. Sometimes, however, she could become a mother hawk, stalking the halls, daring others to mess with her. There were days when we found her warbling away like a songbird by the piano. "They say I have a good voice," she told us in a very private little whisper. At other times, she was a lonely little owl in her big glasses, looking into every face searching for love. When we told her we loved her, she would say, "You do, really? Oh, thank you." She wasn't sure who we were, but she knew she wanted to be loved. She was the bowling wizard of the Alzheimer's ward who sometimes won the tournaments with a little help from the staff. How proud she was when they found a trophy at a garage sale and gave it to her. That symbol sat on her dresser the rest of her life, reminding her that she had worth. Early in her illness, I think she was afraid that she was losing worth, which is a terrible loss. Fortunately, she was surrounded by some very wise caregivers who knew how to love, encourage, and care for these wonderful Alzheimer's souls. I learned so much from them.

We learned to laugh with her about her forgetfulness. It really didn't matter, did it? On the good days, we could make her happy so easily. She was a wonderful advertisement for M&M's, gobbling them down greedily, and a simple treat of a can of root beer thrilled her. It took us a while, but her little social goofs became cherished moments like the time she told my Jewish son-in-law, "You're so tall and good looking. I bet you know how to sing 'The Old Rugged Cross.'"

I can still see her little hand grasping the arm of a waitress when we took her out to dinner. She would keep the waitress talking forever if time and circumstances permitted. Whenever a "captive" would say something, Mother would respond, "Oh really! Well, well, well!" and give a big smile.

"Well, well." I cherish the memory of the cooing sounds she made when she gently held her first great-grandchild in her arms. I cry when I remember her arms outstretched to welcome me, not really knowing who I was. I can now chuckle when I remember the sly winks she would issue in her uninhibited moments.

We all learned to love this Alzheimer's mother. We cherished the shabby red jersey sweater she insisted on wearing, with its ragged sleeves and torn pocket. We learned to give up tormenting her about getting permanents, finding her false teeth, wearing glasses, and all that *silly stuff* that irritated her.

Yes, these were the better memories, the good ones mixed in with the terrible, but returning to the scene I realized that the good memories give those years some meaning. Heartbreak and heart-mend, for in all these memories of my mother one thing comes through: our love for each other. No matter what I had done or said to her during my aggravating adolescence and lifelong thoughtlessness, she had forgiven me and loved me. I find peace now in remembering and chuckling over my funny little Alzheimer's mother, choosing to forget those annoying, suspicious, out-of-hand responses triggered by the disease. Surely I can forgive what she couldn't help.

Strangely enough, my fondest memory is not of the mother I was fortunate to have for all the good years. Rather, I cherish a memory of the mother I see walking away from me down the hall of the nursing home: a stubborn, *almost* 5-foot-tall, self-assured imp, red sweater flapping, one arm swinging, and one hand arrogantly on her hip, head held high. She was *almost* sure of where she was going, boldly daring the world to mess with her. A little hop and skip now and then, the mischief of her showing through. My own personal Charlie Chaplin "Little Bum." I love you, my Alzheimer's Mum. I love you very much.

Our loved ones are not gone until they're gone, and the Alzheimer's years are an important, and often lengthy, part of their lives. A kind of metamorphosis occurs that obscures the person who *was*, but many of us believe that the essence of the person still *is*. I remember when my children were small and would crawl into bed with us on a Sunday morning. I would keep my eyes closed, hoping they would allow me a few more winks. Then I would feel their small fingers prying open my eyelids. "Are you in there, Mommy?" they would inquire. Yes, my mom was still "in there." Those of us who have gone through this to the end know that. The spirit is still alive. Sometimes it is our blindness, and even our rationality, that cannot allow us to be more creative and adaptable in making contact with this precious part of their personality. And sometimes it's because it hurts so much.

FOUR
Developing a Caregiver's Mindset

Do not weep; do not wax indignant.
Understand.

—Baruch Espinoza

Caregiving Is Not Always the Same as Caring

Anyone diagnosed with Alzheimer's will need care. If this person is a member of our family or closely associated, by default, we may end up with the job. Perhaps it is someone we have not been particularly fond of or perhaps it is someone whose dip into dementia is going to tear us apart. Life never warns us in advance which slap in the face we can expect or where it will come from. We just have to cope. Carol explains:

> One of the ironies of this caregiving business is that many of us wind up caring for someone who is not particularly a loved one. Sometimes it's an in-law, sometimes a distant relative, sometimes a parent who was *not kind*. I had this problem. Although deep down I love my mother, I had not liked her for a very long time. In her early stages, I was her major target for anger and frustration. It was hard when she would tell outrageous stories about me to others, and they would believe them because she could appear so normal. I just gritted my teeth and did what I had to do.
>
> Once Mom was placed in a nursing home, her whole personality changed. She became sweet and friendly and very funny. They all loved her. It was all I could do when they would tell me how wonderful it must have been to grow up with someone so funny and charming. I kept my mouth shut with difficulty since my experience was with a mother who was a controlling ———, who treated her husband and children terribly. It is only now, when she is failing, sweet, and helpless, that I have been able to come to terms with

things, and although I can't erase the residual anger and resentment entirely, I can care for her without it.

At some point it is necessary to decide whether you can be comfortable not taking care of this person, whether your conscience or the censure of others will make you feel worse than the caregiving does. Despite the many shining examples of love and care, it is a reality for some that care-GIVING is not always the same as CARING. And for those of you with whom this resounds, it's okay.

If we are honest with ourselves, we are often in a state of panic about taking responsibility for, let alone loving, the Alzheimer's person. Sometimes it's best to acknowledge this right on and find someone else who is better suited to giving the kind of care needed. Some of us are born caregivers, some have practical nursing or other medical training, and some are filled with enough ardor to see it through. Others aren't. It is supreme denial to assume the care of a person in need if we know we just can't do it. On the other hand, if it is possible and we believe that we are up to the task, there are rewards for caregivers. We can find meaning in the giving and, in some instances, long-time hostilities are healed forever. In many instances, great love is shown and great love is received. Let me share Michele's insightful letter:

> Last night I talked with a very old friend, someone who was my teacher when I was twelve, and we've stayed in touch all these many years. I was describing what was happening with my mother and me. And she said I must truly love my parents a lot. I do love them, but explained to her that I thought it was more of a caring for someone who desperately needed someone and that happens to be me.
>
> I was thinking about not having attended church for a number of years when I visited Mom yesterday, but as I was down on my hands and knees putting a clean pair of socks on my mother after her *second* protective underwear change in ten minutes, I thought that it must look like my favorite mass of the Easter season called *The Washing of the Feet*. That is why I do what I do, because of a deep and abiding love. I know I am like so very many of us who love our loved ones in a very special way. I hope this comes across with the humility I feel and is hopefully conveyed.

Why do we do it? Many caregivers take on the task because they love in a very special way. They intuitively know that all of this pain is a part of life that they feel the necessity to share; there is a humility and joy of serving. Sometimes, however, it is just as simple as enjoying the feeling of being needed. Also consider if one has chosen to take such a task, it is considerably less onerous than if one feels forced into it. Like anything else, if we make the commitment and it is not made for us, we can usually see it to a graceful conclusion.

Michele has given us a weighty answer to *the why*, but *the how* is a different problem. What are the secrets to good caring? What roadblocks may keep us from doing a job we can look back on with pride? How can caregivers maintain stability and courage under trying circumstances? Because each family is different and, since all circumstances are just as different, we find there is no *one* way to be a first-class carer. What we can do is offer a few general guidelines.

Avoid Denial

One of the secrets of caring is to face reality. It isn't easy to accept the unacceptable. It is much easier to deny the undeniable. We are prone to close our eyes to the changes in our person because it is too painful to watch. Emotions cloud our sight, and the adrenaline of fear surges through us, obliterating our objectivity.

In *Alzheimer's: A Caregiver's Guide*, Dr. Howard Gruetzner warns:

> Even when family members seem to accept the diagnosis of Alzheimer's disease, denial may leave them vulnerable to shopping for cures or believing that medication prescribed to manage symptoms is really curing the disease.
>
> Sometimes denial re-emerges when there seem to be fluctuations in the person's condition. Good days seem to promise the person is improving. Bad days intensify the family's worries that the person is deteriorating rapidly. Families can profit most by getting off the emotional roller coaster of alternating hope and despair, while making the most of the good days (113).

We deny that Alzheimer's is progressive, and we are elated if our loved one is better just one day. We prepare ourselves for a possible cure or misdiagnosis, only to be socked to the ground when the temporary improvement subsides. Caregivers caught on such a roller coaster are the most susceptible to the lure of snake-oil cures and quick fixes.

Who can blame us for denial? What can we hope for? We can *hope* that our loved one will not suffer. We can *hope* that we can find caring people to help us through this painful experience. We can *hope* that our person is still in there, somewhere. Grasping tightly to our loved one's hand, we cling to the hope of cure even as they teeter precariously toward the downward slope. As one caregiver said when I explained that this book was about the emotions of caregivers, "Oh, I don't think I can read that." We all have a set of blinders and it is irrational to think that they are not sometimes the only protection we have against conclusions we cannot face.

We can deny that the disease is progressive, as Gruetzer warns, but that's not the end of it. There are other varieties of denial. We can deny that the situation our loved one is living in is less than adequate. Keeping a loved one in his or her own home, beyond his or her ability to care for his or her self, is denial. Keeping our loved one with us when we are no longer able to manage is also denial.

We can refuse to look at the toll the disease is taking on *our* health, denying that the caregiving is too much for us. We can deny that others are pushing the brunt of the caregiving on us, not shouldering a fair part of the effort. We can be martyrs to the cause, often to the detriment of our loved one and ourselves. Without wanting to, by turning our blind side, we can be the cause for under- or overmedicating, unsanitary conditions, bedsores, and an inadequate quality of life for all concerned, simply because we refuse to open our eyes to the facts. Either the patient suffers because of inadequate care or the family suffers because of sleep deprivation, stress, burnout, and unspoken feelings of anger or even hate.

If a need for martyrdom, guilt from childhood influences, or an unrealistic view of our own capabilities causes our blindness, this is denial and is harmful to our loved one and to ourselves. We are very ready to complain if a doctor oversteps his or her abilities and refuses to call in a specialist, but we are likely to refuse or be unaware of help and swallow our resentments, our feelings of entrapment, our aching tiredness, depression, anxiety, and emotional exhaustion, turning angrily on others, resenting criticism, and being very disillusioned by the world in general. Time to say "burn out?" Yes.

What determines who should be a caregiver? Age and health of the caregiver for one thing, as well as the number and age of persons in the household must be considered. Is the loved one violent or abusive? What is the health of that person who is giving the majority of care? What is the financial strength of the family and are there finances available to provide adequate outside help? How much respite help in the home can the family afford?

These concerns are what prompted Geri Hall at the University of Iowa, an outstanding leader in the field of Alzheimer's care, to write the following to one caregiver:

Dear _____,

Pease stop for a moment and take a deep breath. I know this is a bit blunt, but several things are very apparent:

1. You love your wife deeply and hate what this disease has done to her.
2. Her agitation became more than you could handle, and it was life-threatening when she was wandering.
3. You are providing total care.
4. You are exhausted.
5. You are conflicted about the medication that maintains her in your home and the desire to maintain your wife medication-free. You want your old wife back.
6. You don't know what to do for conversation or activities for her so the TV is babysitting her. That will soon begin to cause hallucinations so it needs to be replaced ASAP.
7. If you do not get help soon, the stress will quite literally kill you, leaving your wife alone.

I have a couple of suggestions:

1. You need help. No one gets through this disease without outside help. Trust me, it's time. I would strongly recommend a housecleaner, respite so that you can get out for a few hours, and adult day programming.
2. Talk with her doctor about decreasing or changing the medication so that she is less "zombified."
3. Get thee to a support group.
4. Is there a family member who can stay with her while you get some time away?

5. And I know you don't want to hear this, but it is time to start thinking seriously about placement.

Every caregiver comes to a point when he or she makes a clear decision about how many victims the Alzheimer's will take. Please understand that it is time to care for yourself now and let others assume the physical burden of care. If this doesn't happen, you will begin to resent her as much as the disease. As one caregiver said to me, "This weekend I learned just how fine the line is between love and hate."

Please, please take care of yourself.

Geri

When we arrive at this breaking point, as Geri says, we have to decide if we, too, are to be a victim of this disease. We have to ask if we are truly doing the best for our loved one or if we are mechanically going through the motions, too tired and too emotionally frazzled to cope. I know that some of the decisions I made—or neglected to make—for Mother were made when I was too depressed, too tired, and too involved to think straight. Duty and responsibility can drive us far beyond our threshold of endurance. Perfectionists can easily become obsessively focused to the detriment of their health.

But how do we know when we are at the breaking point? (See Appendix C: Caregiver Stress Test.) We may find ourselves unable to focus or organize our thoughts. Perhaps we can't decide what decisions to make or find it too difficult to act upon our decisions. We let things ride. The stress of normal family concerns and the added stress of Alzheimer's can bring on guilt, frustration, and anger, causing us to become combative and belligerent. Deep depression and grief can lead to weight gains, inability to sleep, feelings of inadequacy, a lack of a will to live, and even thoughts of suicide. I can remember a recurring vision of a gun pointed at my head. I honestly didn't feel suicidal, but I sought help nonetheless. It's important to listen to our bodies and pay attention to warning signs. Caregivers are fond of saying, "De Nile is a river in Egypt and must remain there."

Avoid a Sense of Nobodiness

Making my personal return journey awakened me to something else I should have been cognizant of the first time around: the tendency for family members to believe their loved one is no longer there because they are losing their memory. It is natural to look at life and at reason on a continuum of past, present, and future. Someone unable to recognize time concepts or command a once sizeable vocabulary has lost a dimension of human knowledge, and we are apt to give them about as much attention as a snowflake. Here for the moment, but not really present—and not very important.

Early Alzheimer's persons are often aware of the reaction they get from others: dismissive attitudes that minimalize their worth and make them more aware that something terrible and uncontrollable is happening to them. Our body language and subtle expressions are revealing. Understandably, disruptive behavior can result, which makes caregiving even more difficult. It is no wonder that families avoid telling friends and relatives about the disease. No one wants that look of dismissal for his or her loved one.

In her book *Living in the Labyrinth,* Diana Friel McGowin, diagnosed with dementia, explains the plight of the Alzheimer's person. She calls for a right to live, not a right to die and says:

> It is then that I have the worst sense of aloneness and lack of worth. Each one of us must feel they have worth as a living being— a person with the same rights and privileges as the people next door. I feel my lack or worth acutely when I am in large crowds of people. Being in a crowd or even in a busy thoroughfare overwhelms me. All those people "of worth" with places to go. Who knows where they are going? (112).

Add to this the sting of not knowing how much the Alzheimer's loved one knows concerning their disease. Are they afraid? Do they think they're going crazy? Are they eager to ask questions about what is happening to them but afraid that those around them might think them crazy? Do family members wish they would die and get out of everyone's hair? It's a scary, often demeaning kind of mystery game we play in those early days. After Mother died, I found a clue to her silences, her worried look, and her nervous behavior.

The compulsion to secret away small treasures is typical of Alzheimer's, and when Mother was ill, my response to her "squirreling" behavior was amusement or aggravation. When we couldn't find her purse thirty times a day, it was aggravation; when she stuffed bits of this and that into plastic grocery bags and hid them, we were amused.

While searching for items for a family scrapbook last Christmas, I found yet one more of her secret bags, a sad reminder of those terrible days. There it was, tucked in a corner in her old room, just as though some guardian angel had put it there, hoping, perhaps, that now that the stress of caregiving is behind me I would have a better understanding of what Mother went through. In a way, it was a second chance for me.

I tugged at the double knot in the plastic bag and carefully spread the contents in front of me, touching them gently, aware that they had been important to her. I took a moment to look for Mother in these bits of flotsam, and the tears came.

There was an unmailed postcard to her cousin. It was a picture of Bette Davis holding a pillow with the inscription "Old Age Ain't No Place for Sissies." The message on the backside of the card was this: "Dear Fleeta, it was so good for you to write (crossed out) call me. I seem to get more lonesome etc. etc. every day. I saw this card and I thought at least we aren't sissies! We have to have a laugh once . . . " *Message* not finished. Card not mailed. Alzheimer's amnesia strikes again.

She had included two or three greeting cards from friends with pictures and notes tucked inside. Were they there to remind her she still had friends? There were also two notes in my father's handwriting. One read, "Sweetie, Gone to 27th Street. B back soon. Take you to dinner. Love, Me." She had included someone's note of condolence from my father's funeral. Here was a list of her pledges paid to her church, as well as a feared Medicare bill with lots of underlining, reminding me how afraid she was of unpaid bills.

In addition, there was a picture of some people I never knew, two florist bills, a small notepad, *four* copies of medicines she was taking, and *four* repetitions of what each medicine was supposed to accomplish, reminders of reminders of reminders. Obviously she was trying desperately to remember the most important things, and yet she had said nothing to me.

My fingers picked at the pieces, not sure what to make of them, lingering at the saddest note of all—a small scrap of paper torn from a yellow pad. Mother had written: "Sing—Cross to Bear—, Psychosea, de-mentia–mind is–brain is losing part cells. Cells."

In the midst of this hellish disease, Mother had obviously known that something was happening to her, and she wanted to know what it was. "Phychosea, dementia," she called it. "Sing," she had written. Did she think that she could sing away the fear and loneliness and make it go away? "Rock of Ages, cleft for me." I ache when I think of her solitude. I remember her standing sadly at the back door staring outside, but only later did I realize the pain of her loneliness and fear.

Even if I had known the isolation she felt, I lacked the talents or knowledge that might have healed that broken soul. I could not heal her, lonely and crying out for those she had loved. I know she also cried for the blankness she could feel commanding her to bow down before it. Is it always so? She cried to "go home" and I couldn't help. She had packed her little plastic bag, ready to go, but couldn't find her way. Is it always so?

Are we always this alone when we come face-to-face with our own life-threatening pain? Could she have faced anything worse than aware-ness of her own dementia, afraid to confide in friends and family while clinging desperately to some semblance of control, that tight knot in a plastic bag? Is it always so?

Even in the terrible confusion of losing "those cells," Mother had cir-cled one sentence inside a used sympathy card. I rescued it from the bag. It read, "Lo, I am with you always." Out of the pit comes the child: faithful, hopeful, and "of such is the kingdom of heaven." She had found her own way.

Survival With Dignity

For the sake of everyone concerned, it is important to preserve hope. Hope does not necessarily indicate denial. It is just hope. New research and experimental methods of retraining the mind are currently in the scientific pipeline and the controversy continues. Can you reverse Alz-heimer's symptoms? The experts have yet to agree. So until that time comes, let's be realistic but not close-minded or undereducated. Morris, diagnosed with Alzheimer's in 1998, awakens us to an Alzheimer's fu-ture with more promise:

When I was first diagnosed with Alzheimer's, I didn't think Martin Luther King, Jr. had anything personally to say to me. Nature was to blame, not society, and wasn't society doing all it could for people like me? Just like it was "doing all it could" for a black kid who was advised to get a job as a janitor because he didn't even use the word 'be' correctly—you can't argue with biology!

But then I started learning about the opportunities for rehabilitation, at least occasionally, available to persons with other brain disorders, all kinds of brain disorders, as long as they weren't labeled "progressive" and "incurable." I reread King's magnificent Letter from a Birmingham Jail, where he passionately spoke out about the indignities and terrors of being a southern black, and a phrase jumped out at me. " . . . when you are forever fighting a degenerating sense of nobodiness . . ." What a perfect description of what we're up against.

The American Dream, for which King died, is that nobody deserves to feel "a degenerating sense of nobodiness." Everybody needs an opportunity to develop his or her potential to the fullest. We who have Alzheimer's can struggle for this dream to become a reality. We can learn from King and his movement. We can boldly face the worst and in the teeth of it proclaim we are still *Somebody*, because of the Truth of Something beyond our losses. Then we can fight for an America where every disabled person can sit in the front of the bus![1]

Morris gives us something else to think about. Alzheimer's Associations around the world should aspire to a new paradigm: dementia survival with dignity. We are claiming our full participation in cultural life and thus making a stand for all persons with cognitive limitations.

> *The Sun of love can pierce the cognitive fog.*
> *As normal people we are taught, perhaps*
> *wrongly to put our emotions aside in*
> *order to be as rational as possible, but*
> *when we become demented we must*
> *lovingly gather them together.*
> —Morris, living with Alzheimer's

Who can say it better? Our person is with us until death and "survival with dignity" should be our indispensable mantra. So many caregivers decry the loss of dignity in this disease. We hesitate to admit it, but we often feel embarrassed by the lack of inhibitions left to our loved one.

We are dumbfounded by the kind of irrational things they may do. If we truly believe this is unacceptable, one of our major tasks should be to educate others and ourselves about the dignity that lies just below the surface. We know that our father, mother, husband, or wife is still there somewhere, and that their personhood involves more than their memory. We have much to learn about dementia, but we're beginning to discover a few tools to help us communicate.

Barbara has been a caregiver for a long time and she says:

> Sure is a weird disease and difficult for those of us used to being problem solvers. There is no thread of continuity, no rationalizing the irrational, nothing relating to anything. The best lesson and the most helpful for me was to learn (as soon as possible) that every moment is just every moment, and live in it with your loved one the best you know how.

Every moment is just every moment, a wise way to give care.

The Minefields of Non-Reason

Everything that is rational in us resists the steps we take in order to connect with our Alzheimer's loved one. "Three little men visited me last night." "Alice, I have to tell you, your husband stole my doll collection." To argue with the reality of the Alzheimer's person is useless. Seems that sometimes the loved one can remember these hallucinations when he or she cannot remember his or her own name. Your husband may not be welcome in your mother's home for months if she really believes the tale of the doll theft. Probably she has carefully stored the collection somewhere and forgotten where it is.

Certain things help communication and other things don't. Each of us has to discover our own path through the mind tangles if there is to be any peace. "Don't worry, I'll take care of it," I often told Mother and saved, "I love you. Would I let something like that happen to you?" for her headiest illusions. Distraction works for many, a candy treat for others. You will find that certain techniques work all of the time and some of them work, but only sometimes.

Even in her wildest Alzheimer's-ridden minutes, Mother could always find my most vulnerable spot and send in a quick reprimand. "Have you ever been here before to visit me?" "Oh, I didn't think I had any family." "You think you're so smart. I bet you're poisoning me." "Look at this old rag I'm wearing." (An old red sweater no one could get off of her!) We are convinced that not only are our loved ones present, but that Alzheimer's is bringing out the qualities we liked least in them. At these times you can only grit your teeth and keep repeating, "It's the disease talking. It's the disease talking."

Gifted caregiving requires creativity, it requires us to be on our toes twenty-four hours a day. Here's how Nancy learned to adapt:

> I remember one time I drove her to the doctor and when I pulled up in front of the building she asked where we were. I said, "At the doctor's." She said, loudly and argumentatively, "This isn't the place. This ISN'T my doctor's!" I pulled out, drove around the block, and when we pulled up again in front of the same building, I said, "Here we are, Mom! At the right place." She looked at me and said, "Now THIS is the place."
>
> Many times I save the day with a walk out of the room. If she wouldn't wear a particular article of clothing, I'd walk out, walk back in, and say, "Gee, Mom, I was thinking that your red jacket would be really great with that blouse." Sure enough, she'd agree.
>
> I wish you tons of creativity and patience, a continuing strong spirit, and warm friends to love and hug you.

At the same time there are moments of pure magic. Consider the art exhibited in the Alzheimer's Association's "Memories in the Making"[2] program. The creativity remaining within the Alzheimer's person is amazing. Somehow the emotional, the artistic, musical, and instinctual moments are greater with Alzheimer's patients after the disease sets in. As inhibitions fail, they are replaced by a freedom of spirit that can be disconcerting but also very beautiful. At this point an Alzheimer's mind can resemble a white jigsaw puzzle. We don't know what to expect and they don't know what to expect. The results can be awesome, inspiring, and thought-provoking. Yes, it keeps us on our toes.

The Simple Pleasure of Giving

When we are faced with the real probability of caregiving, we have to ask ourselves, "Are we a caregiver?" I worried, fretted, and wrung my hands hard enough to have won some sort of prize, but I now see the futility and error of the worrywart face I assumed with the onset of Mother's disease. Emily is the owner of a caring Alzheimer's assisted-living facility. She shares a professional's point of view:

> I see it so often with the residents in my homes. There are some whose families stay devoted and involved and others where, except for the obligatory visit, they keep their distance. I have come to believe that some people have no idea how to handle illness in others—and probably in themselves as well. I have also come to realize that to maintain a relationship with someone with Alzheimer's requires that you really do understand, in a very deep way, that giving is receiving. People often look at what they get out of a relationship in a very, very narrow way. I try to help people see that to reach out across the barrier of Alzheimer's, you can have moments that are as deep and meaningful as any one will ever have. I also think that most people constantly see what they no longer have or what is no longer there, instead of focusing on the simple pleasure of giving.
>
> There is a daughter of one of my residents who visits regularly and brings her children. She comes with no expectations. Her mother is very advanced, but when her mother sits still, she talks to her, touches her, and kisses her when she can. She encourages her children to talk to her as well. Every so often the grandmother will brighten up and smile. That is its reward.
>
> The daughter once said that even though her mother may not be in a mood to take what they have to give, she is aware that her visits mean something to the other residents. It is obvious how much she loves and respects her mother, and the disease has not altered that.

Dr. Janice Lessard, an internist-geriatrician in Toronto, has been working with seniors since 1967. She gives us another view of the caregiver:

> In my experience, caregivers who are laid back, with a sense of humor, last the longest. Carers who are perfectionists, worrywarts, and/or alarmists don't last very long at all. These characteristics are often totally independent of the degree or type of needs of dependent seniors.

What keeps a good caregiver going? Sometimes it only a prayer that a glimmer of the loved one's personality may surface. We call these precious moments *"windows."*

Windows

Geri Hall admits to "mysteries" in this disease that fascinate her scientific mind:

> Windows of lucidity and flashes of transient memory are a mystery to us all. They make the disease frustrating, fascinating, and cause us to re-examine our beliefs about the brain, spirituality, and the nature of disease. I think of them somewhat poetically—like crocuses in the snow—reminding us that the person is still there, inside, somehow knowing. I know I'm supposed to be a "scientist," but there are times when the mysteries are sweeter.

They call them windows. The brain opens for a moment, it breathes a fresh breath of air from somewhere, and your loved one is back. But only for the moment. When it does happen, it's usually early in the disease. Those moments are so joyful. They are our reward and our undoing. They hurt so much, but they help us remember that our person is still there. As we practice our carer skills it helps to know that if we're aware, we may see a glimpse of the person we remember.

I was heartbroken to see my mother's personality extinguished, but ever so gently, now and again, she would return, a memory in a smile, a teasing look, or an astute question intelligently phrased. She would grasp my hand with that conspiratorial look, and we were best buddies once more. She would speak to her great-grandchild in the universal tongue of womanhood, cooing and holding him to her shoulder, never missing a step. She would cry tears for my dad, now dead several years. Then the curtain would fall again and she was gone.

It really takes very little to make a carer happy. My friend, Sarah, wrote me about these windows during her husband's illness:

> The windows I spoke to you about, three of them, occurred in the first year after diagnosis. The first was dramatic, starting about noontime when it was very apparent he was totally with it. He asked questions about why he was taking medicines, what strange things he was doing, why didn't he remember any of these things, where had we gone to see doctors, and what they said. Then he looked at me and said, "My God, you've been going through hell!" Oh, thank you God for letting him know and telling me, I thought. When I

asked him what it seemed like to him, he said there were "holes in his brain" with unconnected pieces of information. He frantically began to write down a chronology of events so he'd know what had gone on. After about six hours he gradually faded—that's the best word I can find—until he was confused, anxious, aggressive, and my John was once again hidden.

I, of course, thought that the diagnosis was a mistake, but the doctor explained. "These are windows. We know the information is there, but just can't be accessed." I thought, "Sure that's all you know about it." The next window opened for about two hours, and he again wrote down all the events and then answered a phone call from a friend in Connecticut. I could see he was beginning to lose it. He couldn't quite grasp the conversation nor remember just what had been said.

The last time was only about a half-hour and he didn't have the clarity even of the first two. These events, and the fact that even now bits of intelligence will surface, have convinced me that John is still inside the shell of his body, but can't, on a consistent basis, access his personal files. All along I have described his disease as a computer and been laughed at, but initially, if he couldn't access the information one way, I could get him to find it by going another route. For example, if I said, "We're going to the grocery store," he couldn't reason that out. But if I said something like, "We'll take the car and go down the road by the highway," then he would know instantly what and where I was talking about. Or if I said, "Let's go to the river," he'd be mixed up, but if I said, "Let's go out back and through the trees until we get down there," then he'd know.

As I reread this it sounds as though it is a lack of noun recognition, but it wasn't that. It was access. I think he had to get around a "hole." So in my heart of hopes, I think the brain isn't all destroyed and maybe someday something will help restore the connections.

Wishful thinking? Possibly. The best we can do is care for our loved ones with dignity and love, trying to be realistic about the disease but suspending reality, when necessary, to protect the spirit. With a giving heart and a sense of humor, perhaps we can make their lives as happy and safe as humanly possible. Perhaps we can take some of the stress from ourselves, if we live each moment as it comes and pray for a "window."

And so, we repeat:

Do not weep; do not wax indignant. Understand.

FIVE
Day by Day with the Stranger

Morris, diagnosed with Alzheimer's, reveals his outlook regarding his future:

> I find the Serenity Prayer invaluable. "God, grant me the serenity to accept the things I cannot change, the courage to change the things I can, and the wisdom to know the difference." Acceptance comes first. "One day at a time" helps too. Maybe tomorrow I will forget everything I've learned and done today, but God will remember.
>
> I think the reason that I can use myself as a guinea pig is that I have the courage to risk failure. And because prayers for courage are sometimes answered.

We can read all the helpful books on the subject and attend all the advanced Alzheimer's educational seminars in the world, but when it comes to daily hands-on care, there is no one there but the caregiver and the loved one. While others may offer sympathy, advice (lots of that), criticism, and an occasional visit, no one but the caregiver wipes the chin, cleans up the messes, and protects this Alzheimer's stranger; and no one else can protect his or her dignity and courage. In any given family there is generally one person, or perhaps two, who assume the daily responsibility, and as the disease progresses this becomes twenty-four/seven.

We can discuss all of the esoteric ideas about what Alzheimer's care *should* be, but the day-to-day care is an exercise in anticipation and frustration. If we could predict what we will have to muddle through next, we would have it made. But, because we are usually one step, or better yet, one symptom, behind the disease, we are forever unable to catch up, and bedlam reigns. It's a rocky road. Whenever I consider just how difficult caregiving is, I am amazed that seventy-five percent of Alzheimer's patients are cared for at home.

"One can't believe impossible things."
"I daresay you haven't had much practice,"
said the Queen. "When I was your age,
I always did it for half an hour a day.
Why sometimes I've believed as many as
six impossible things before breakfast."
—Lewis Carroll, *Through the Looking Glass*

The Behinder Type

Unfortunately, I always felt that I was the "behinder" type. I seemed to be behind in searching for help, in finding creative solutions to problems, and in taking care of myself. I had been engaged in the tasks of raising kids, teaching school, and making a home. My world of rationality was not prepared for the loop-de-loop we had to take with Mother's illness.

I recently found a journal that I tried to keep while Mother was still at home. Reading it over, I thought, "Oh, my! How does one cope with this?" I really didn't cope. I was just kind of was "there," slack jawed and dumbfounded, not knowing which hole Alice and I had jumped into. It shows what we were going through at the time and brings up some questions. Could I have done a better job? Yes, if I had known more, known where to go for help, and if I had been able to anticipate what was to come, but as I said, I was a "behinder."

Here are a few excerpts from my journal:

> May 13, Mother's Day
>
> At 5:30 P.M. Mother is fine and just great at 6 P.M. Then about 8 P.M., we heard a noise in the laundry room and found her frantically rolling out a tube of Cling Free.
>
> "I'm starving to death," she said, searching frantically for food in the Cling Free. That was hard to believe because she'd had a full dinner followed by two candy bars. We gave her more cookies and tried to understand what was happening. "Did Estelle and Spike come yet?" she wanted to know. I answered that Spike was upstairs. "No, that's the dog," she remembered correctly. She was looking for her cousin and her husband, Spike, who lived 1,000 miles away. At 10 P.M. she fell asleep.

At 10:30 P.M. Mother came upstairs saying, "I have to use the bathroom." She had forgotten that there was one downstairs next to her bedroom. After using the bathroom, she seemed to settle down. I checked on her, found her asleep with her glasses still perched on her nose. I took them off, afraid she would fall and hurt herself as she had once before. I looked down and saw that she had used a silk scarf to tie an old school bell to her wrist. When I asked her the next morning why she had done this, she said she wanted to be sure she woke up if she got out of bed. This is the mystery of Alzheimer's: at one moment lost in another world, and yet still aware that what she is doing isn't quite right. Sometimes all we can do is shake our heads.

June 23

At 4 P.M. Mother is confused. She lost her purse (Oh, Lordy! That purse!) and at 5 P.M. she refuses to stop walking. "I have to get things ready for church." At 5:15 P.M. she is putting her shoes, bra, and panties in a paper sack. Foolishly, I tried to get her to stop walking and received a motherly scolding as my reward. Between 5 P.M. and 3 A.M. she is:

- Upstairs with watermelon and bananas, rummaging in our bookcase, purse on her arm, stuffing the fruit in between Leon Uris and Shakespeare.
- Downstairs, where she fell over a table and chairs. I caught her and she runs to look under the stairway for food. This insane hunger!
- Shaking me awake to tell me she lost $200 in a basket and needs to get it "before the crowds come."
- In our bathroom looking for food and her purse.
- Up at 1 A.M. getting ready for church. She asks me, "Didn't we go to the country yesterday?"
"No, we were here all day."
"Well, the man at the home said, "You just don't have anyone, do you?" We were never able to identify man or home, but he showed up quite often as a source of great wisdom.

There were various references to my husband and myself separately about her loneliness. At times I am her mother and at other times I am a distrusted stranger.

Mother sundowned regularly. Sundowning is the term given to the extreme agitation, anxiety, and even hallucinations that occur late in the afternoon or in the early evening. The phenomenon is poorly under-stood but is thought to be triggered by fatigue or anxiety. One particu-larly bad evening Mother disassociated and thought she was in Indiana, when actually we were in Colorado. We tried to reason with her, telling her that all her things were right here but her answer was, "All these things are copies of my things." She began packing her Bible and her mother's Bibles into her plastic bags, telling us, "The man in the hall said I am getting the wrong medicine."

When I suggested calling her doctor, she violently shook a tiny fin-ger at me, claiming that she would die if I called the doctor, and "There will be proof that you have changed my medicines." Her excuse for not going to bed was that she had to go home. "I need my purse so I can go home." Commenting on her furniture she told us, "All these things are old, and the first time I ever saw them was in a dime store in a special display."

Like a movie running backwards, dementia leaves the watcher dumb-struck with disbelief. Why was she so hungry? I knew she was lonely and yet what could we do about that? Why was she turning night into day? Do Alzheimer's patients enact their dreams? Why did she distrust me? I felt hurt. Other than tell little white lies as a child, I had never done anything to make my mother doubt me. Well, almost never.

As I go through my old diary, I see things more clearly than I did at that time. Poor mother was a ship without a rudder, and I was totally unprepared to be caught in the middle of her dementia storm. I had no idea how to cope, no education, and no experience. Now I can see the mistakes I made that made it harder for my mother and me:

- I tried to reason with her when there was no reason.
- We had no help in caring for her. I now know one cannot do this alone.
- I didn't recognize sundowning; it was a complete puzzle to me. Now I would know not to let her get overtired, drink coffee, or get stressed late in the day.
- I argued with her. What a waste of time!
- I took her paranoid comments personally. I honestly thought she must mean these terrible things she was saying. Now I know it was the disease talking.
- I was uptight and had misplaced my sense of humor.

Dealing with Helter-Skelter

When one is going through a storm, it is tough to keep to the high peaks or take refuge in the low ground. The whirling winds often seem to be coming from all directions, too hard and fast for us to gain a foothold. If you read over Mother's comments you begin to sense the helter-skelter nature of her Alzheimer's and of our lives during this period. Ricocheting from one idea to another, from paranoia to visual bewilderment, and on to a waking dream world in the space of few minutes, she left any rational person struggling to catch up. There was no order. There was no logic. There was no way to logically handle the situations that arose. We can deal with it here, encapsulated in the lexicon of the disease. This, in itself, lends logic. But day-to-day caregiving takes the unreasoning genie out of the bottle, casting spells on us and those we love both in daylight and darkness. There is no box, no boundaries, no handles to grab hold of.

Sherry is caught between the illogic of the situation and important family concerns as her mother's paranoia becomes worse:

> My mom will be eighty-six in June. One of the problems I am having is dealing with the delusions she has been having lately. Of course they are real to her. Unfortunately, instead of thinking that her dead brother is alive, her delusions are all negative. A biggie lately is that my husband is beating me. Although it's not true and there is no reason for her to think this, when she has this thought in her head there is no convincing her otherwise.
>
> Another example is that after seeing her this weekend, I talked to her the next day and she was mad at me because she said I left her in an angry mood about something. Again this isn't true and there's no basis for her even to have such a thought. There have been others, too; she thinks my brother is in jail among other things. Are there medications to help this problem?

Something is needed here. Sherry and her husband cannot expect to have a happy home life if her mother is there ready to scream at her son-in-law whenever he enters the house, or if she is dredging up angry thoughts about her daughter on a regular basis. This may be the time to ask the doctor for a medication or, if the atmosphere is threatening their marriage, it may be time to consider different living arrangements for her mother. No one wants it that way, but the lives of all concerned are important and must be considered.

Frustrating Decision-Making

Philosopher Soren Kirkegaard said, "I see it all perfectly; there are two possible situations—one can either do this or that. My honest opinion and my friendly advice is this: do it or do not do it—you will regret both." Nowhere is this truer than in Alzheimer's care.

Anyone connected with this disease will agree. The decisions one makes with Alzheimer's all seem wrong. There are no good answers, no good decisions. Many times you are unable to make your loved one happy. Other times you're limited in your choices by family, money issues, or even religious constraints. One's own ability or inability to give care limits our choices, and lack of support from the government or institutional officials stands in our way. Our choices are always limited by the knowledge that this disease will win and any decision we make will seem wrong. All decisions are only the best of the available alternatives. Always there are limits. Sometimes the only answer is to say:

Yes, I'll Cry

Each day I watch my mother walk,
I hear her sigh, I hear her talk.
She speaks of loved ones no longer here.
I watch helpless, as she sheds a tear.
Alzheimer's is stealing my mother away,
And she grows worse each passing day.
She needs help with all her care,
From getting dressed to brushing her hair.
We cut her food to help her eat.
This once tidy woman is no longer neat.
She often seems to live in the past,
Please dear God, how long will this last?
As her memory goes, I can only stand by,
Frustrated and helpless, and yes, . . . I cry.
Those who love her, she no longer knows.

How long till her memory completely goes?
Each day I watch my mother walk.
I hear her sigh, I hear her talk.
I watch daily as she slowly dies,
I can't help her, and yes, I cry.
—Jerry Ham, Caregiver and Son

But, grown men don't cry, do they?
Unless they happen to have a loved one with
something like Alzheimer's disease, and then,
MAYBE it's okay—once in a while.
—Bill, Caregiver and Husband

There is a time for tears. Sometimes nothing else helps, and sometimes there is no other answer.

However, Peter, who lives in Boston, gives us a slap in the face and an eye-opening look at the decisions we will have to make. His mother's illness became a great learning and sharing experience for him, and his personal pain comes through in his message. Listen carefully, for Peter has been able to help many caregivers with his "no nonsense" approach to caregiving:

I'm sorry if I don't look at everything as sunshine and flowers. If you want to know about AD, then know about it. To know is also to accept the rage, the anger, and the passion: to accept the pain and suffering on both sides, to love, to hate. It is compassion, love, and caring. It is also fighting and doing what you have to do to care for your loved one. You can put it in nice cute little packages, or you can deal with it.

By not dealing with central issues, I hope and pray they do not consume you. If not already, you will be faced with legal and Medicare problems. You will face problems with denial, exhaustion, good and bad doctoring, and good and bad nursing-home care. You may face being a part of the sandwich generation, caring for parents and children. You will be exposed to watching one spouse kill himself or herself in caring for another. You will see neglect, bad medicating, bad diagnosis, and the problems of secondary conditions. Nursing homes that should be boarded up or burnt down, people who should be barred from medicine, who may have been censured, but you will never know. You will find children, parents, outreach people, doctors, nurses, and support people who deserve sainthood. You will also meet the same people who deserve time in jail.

Your references and paperwork will fill a small office. You will, if you have not already, chase down three years of your parents' paperwork. You will have to know your parent's rights under the law. You will likely become guardian or POA.[1]

As dementia sets in you will become their agent in order to protect their rights. You will listen to snake-oil salesmen telling you about the magic cure that doesn't exist. You will have to learn a million different ways to lie on cue because you love someone. You will feel guilt like you have never felt it in your life.

And, if you allow it, you will never find a greater love than you have ever experienced. You will have to decide to be a proactive advocate or sit and watch laws that will take away more from your loved one than has already been taken. These are real day-to-day Alzheimer's issues.

Peter accepted the care of his mother with an emotion and passion that few of us extend, and yet, somehow, because of his desire to wage war on her behalf, he gained a kind of peace and reward for his brusque, man-like service. Unable to work and still care for his mother at home, Peter placed her in a Catholic nursing home. He worried about the placement and when everything seemed to be going fairly well, he wrote:

> Mom did a total turn around at St. Pat's: people all the time, activities, and ice cream. I let her (and myself) adjust a few weeks and she did splendidly. She is very tiny with severe osteoporosis and scoliosis. So she's cute—what can I say? We walk hand-in-hand, the odd couple. We have become closer. In another ironic twist, I have always wanted to have closeness to my mom. It was through this disease that love and caring manifested themselves. We are both blessed. She is safe, well-protected, and loved. I couldn't ask for more.

Get Along and Go Along

One way to ease the suffering of daily care is to develop a "get along, go along" attitude. It cuts down on casualties. Carlene has learned to accept her father's reality:

Even though my Dad has been in a confused state for a few years now, every now and then I find myself trying to reason with him. Take last night for example. He refused to go to bed, and by about 5 A.M. I stomped into the garage and demanded that he get out of the truck and go to bed. Remember everyone, this is the man that runs naked through the neighborhood and picks all my green tomatoes every chance he gets. Needless to say, I have been sitting up with him all night. My patience was wearing a little thin by this time. In a gruff voice I said, "What is wrong with you? Why can't you just listen to me and go to bed?"

He gave me one of his looks like, "What's your problem, lady?" and went back to sticking a piece of cord in the ignition of the truck. I realized then that I am the one who knows what is wrong with him. He has no idea that anything is wrong with him. For a minute there, I lost it and tried to force him to face reality. We all know that this does not work and for the most part, only makes things worse, but we all continue to try to make them understand, for some reason.

My point is that even though I know better and have "accepted" my dad's world as his reality, I sometimes slip back to the old me and try to bring him into the real world. It never works, and I hope that someday soon I will stop trying. Life is so much easier for both of us if we stay in "his world."

Life *is* smoother if we can stay in the Alzheimer's world. It also helps relieve some of the frustration in communicating. A caregiver friend shares a story about her father-in-law:

One of the lessons we have learned in dealing with my father-in-law and his particular manifestations of mental impairment is how to ask a question. We will never ever allow a health care professional to ask him a yes or no question again. When we saw a second doctor to get him some pain relief, my father-in-law responded "no" to every question he asked, including "Does your back hurt?" It was infuriating because the doctor can't treat him for pain if he says there is none.

Well, the exact same thing happened with the anesthesiologist. The doctor explained the test results, why he was hurting, and described the procedure for the injections. Then he asked Dad, "Are you ready to proceed with the injections?" You guessed it. "No!" My husband accompanied him on that visit. The doctor couldn't do the injections when Dad said he didn't want them. I ended up phoning the doctor, asking him to rephrase the question so Dad would have to make a statement rather than say yes or no. The doctor then asked him, "What would you like me to do?" And Dad said, "Give me the shots." Whew!

I think this is important for others to understand. My father-in-law really had pain and really wanted the injections. But, when it comes to answering a yes or no question, all he can say is "no." I don't know why this is, but it is.

Getting him to "describe the pain" or anything that requires a complete statement is better than asking a yes or no question. However, I did make up flash cards over the weekend with the word "yes" on them. I told him that we were going to learn a new word this weekend. He said, "What word?" And I flashed the card: Y—E—S.

Creative Problem Solving

We have to be just as creative or even more so in dealing with some of the more serious daily problems of Alzheimer's care: wandering, driving, safety issues, and problems with bathing, medicating, and feeding; none of these issues are easily resolved. We dare not take a "get along, go along" approach with these. Too much is at stake.

Wandering, for example, *must* be stopped. Each year many Alzheimer's patients never return home. We have to register our loved ones with Safe Return[2] through the Alzheimer's Association and we need to provide safety locks or alarms to prevent their leaving home. There is no "get along" attitude about this. The percentage of wandering dementia patients returned to their homes greatly increases if they are properly tagged for identity recognition.

To say, "Well, he only wandered once," or to criticize and cringe at the locked door policy of many Alzheimer's units displays a lack of understanding of this disease. Casual observers do not understand that in some ways Alzheimer's patients become like small children, and yet we would not allow a three-year-old to wander about town. We have to find ways of protecting with dignity, but they *must* be protected.

Driving is another difficult issue for families, maybe one of the most difficult. Our loved ones are more apt than others their age to have accidents or get lost and perhaps never find their way home. On the one hand, we hesitate to curtail their freedom, and still we know they should not be on the streets. Yet driving is almost an American birthright, and to remove that privilege can be downright devastating. The loved one may not be able to remember almost anything, but chances are they will remember the anger they feel toward the person who takes away their driving privileges.

To do this means facing the reality of what can happen, like an accident in which one's loved one or someone else is injured or killed or a civil lawsuit in which the family is held to blame because they allowed a demented person behind the wheel. Driving must be monitored and finally curtailed. Families may have to file down keys, enlist the aid of doctors, and/or get rid of cars to stop this dangerous activity. However, if we are to do it with dignity, it means being sure that other means of transportation are available. We cannot leave a loved one trapped in a home without the ability to run errands and occasionally see people. Families can share this duty or enlist the aid of local transportation opportunities for seniors. Call your local transportation service or contact the Alzheimer's Association.

Bathing requires us to provide for modesty and flexibility of schedules. He or she may not need a bath every day, and rigid scheduling may not be the answer to cooperation. Some things aren't worth the fight. If you see a battle looming, schedule the bath for tomorrow and provide a warm, cozy environment when you do suggest it the next time.

Do what I didn't do. The Alzheimer's Association, the Alzheimer's Society in Canada, and many other Alzheimer's organizations have information and ideas on all the activities of daily living: bathing, eating, taking medications, activities, and so on. I just didn't ask.

Energizer Bunnies

Mother always reminded me of the Energizer bunny her last few years. Heart problems and other complaints seemed to fade into the background as Alzheimer's took the forefront. We were fortunate enough to have a wonderful activity director in Mother's Alzheimer's wing. The residents sang, they bowled, they had their nails painted. They did everything imaginable.

Most Alzheimer's patients need activity. Without it, like small children, they get into all sorts of trouble. This is not well-understood by some caregivers and facilities. What is the benefit of placing a loved one in an Alzheimer's-specific unit? Unlike the general population of a nursing home, Alzheimer's patients are usually in fairly good physical health. Without activity, boredom, depression, and aggressive behavior may occur. Pam shows us the way she keeps her mother active:

> I did best with Mother's nervous and compulsive symptoms by doing something more active with her like having her sweep the carport or go for a long walk in the neighborhood or mall. All of these activities were designed to wear her out, which they did. By the time we got back, there were fewer nervous and compulsive symptoms. If I could get her focused on her coloring book, the rubbing back and forth of the colored pencil seemed to help.
>
> Altering a few things in the house helped. She constantly wanted to water and handle the artificial arrangements in the den on a plant rack. I finally admitted defeat and moved them to another room. I put plants there that could live in water and let her water to her heart's content. She wasn't being told no, and I wasn't going crazy. She also rubbed the grain of the wood on a wooden TV tray and counter desk in the kitchen. I finally gave her the same TV tray and let her ruin it, but it was easily replaceable compared to an end table or dining room table. I put a piece of glass over the wooden kitchen desk. She rubbed and rubbed all she wanted, and it didn't do anymore damage.

Another resolution to the activity need is the adult day care center. It is a very welcome addition to the resources in our community that have proliferated in the last ten years; some are even dementia-specific. They will, for a sum of money, provide care, lunch, and activities for your loved one, and some provide physical activities and field trips for high-functioning Alzheimer's patients. Many of these are excellent resources and have played a major role in families' ability to keep their loved ones at home for a longer time. Some are even able to care for patients overnight, allowing caregivers to get a weekend break now and then.

Loss of Inhibitions

One of the most difficult things to accept is that, as the disease progresses, the inhibitions of a lifetime are lost. We don't *inherently* have good table manners or sexual considerations. These are learned responses. We have learned to say the correct thing in a polite conversation, we bathe in order to keep ourselves from smelling, and we have found our way to the bathroom countless times since our mothers taught us to.

As the Alzheimer's person leaves "civilization" so to speak, many learned behaviors are lost. A loved one may eat with his or her fingers, stuffing food into his or her face at a furious rate or even eating things that are harmful. A friend's husband had a taste for Brillo pads. Some patients, in later stages, need to be watched like naughty two-year-olds to keep them from consuming the cleaning supplies under the sink. Table manners and language may sink to a new low at certain stages and it is tempting to try to protect our loved one from social contact or, perhaps, we really want to protect ourselves and the social contact from the loved one. Mother would accompany us to a movie and snore loudly, disturbing everyone I'm sure. But she loved the trip, and a nudge in the ribs usually woke her for a period of time.

One of the most distressing behaviors to caregivers is incontinence. It is not the ordinary incontinence of the mentally alert aging person. This is the incontinence of someone who uses a wastebasket at night. This is the incontinence of someone who will eat feces, wave diapers, and urinate on kitchen cabinets or in corners. It is no surprise that three-fourths of ALL patients in nursing homes are incontinent. It is one of the most difficult daily problems for caregivers to deal with.

In the summer of 1995, the national newsletter of the Alzheimer's Association reported on other difficult Alzheimer's behaviors:

> Some of the more distressing sexual expressions exhibited by individuals with Alzheimer's may include paranoid thoughts about secret relationships; misidentification of a partner; inappropriate advances toward others, bold or lewd behavior; and hypersexuality.

In the same article is this idea:

> "It's hard to be a caregiver and a lover." Debra Cherry, Ph.D., clinical psychologist and associate executive director of the Los Angeles chapter of the Alzheimer's Association, explains that this is common. "Adults can enjoy satisfying relationships later in life . . . but for many Alzheimer couples, loss of intimacy becomes another major casualty of the disease"(Advances 8–9).

Acknowledging the problem and discussing it with experts are probably the best things to do, but sexual behaviors nonetheless represent a particularly difficult and private problem. While the patient is unaware of his or her actions, the family is acutely discomfited. Sarah's husband removed his wedding ring and tried to flush it down the toilet. He accompanied that with close relationships with some of the female patients in the nursing home and jealousies developed whenever my friend would visit. Sarah tried not to let it bother her, but at a time when she saw him leaving her mentally, this sexual attraction to other women was tough to accept. He seemed to be retreating from her in every possible way.

Julie's story shows just how troubling, if harmless, a patient's escapades can be:

> They called from the nursing home. "Julie, we found your mother in bed with Mr. Fred."
>
> "Mr. Fred?" I did a quick double take. Mr. Fred was about four feet tall and not my idea of anybody's sexual dreamboat!
>
> "Yes, she was guiding his hand . . ."
>
> My mother? Miss Manners? I picked my chin off the floor and "intelligently" replied, "Well, what should we do about it?"
>
> The director of the unit tried to educate me to the fact that sexual incidents are common among Alzheimer's patients. I dumbly listened as she explained, not really listening. All I could think of was, "MY mother? Mr. Fred? You've got to be kidding!" Like a protective parent, I was ready to go over and throttle Mr. Fred, except I was about twice his size and it would have been no match.
>
> So, here's where the younger generation helps out. I quickly dialed my daughter, having to share this new bit of trauma with her. "Lisa, they found Grandma in bed with a MAN!" I gasped.
>
> "So?" Was my daughter's reply. (*She's* cool). "Mom, if they can have a little pleasure, what difference does it make?"

Yes, Alzheimer's teaches us to see life painted in different colors than we ordinarily view it. Some things just don't matter. We have more important things to consider: how to get medicines into a stubborn mother, how to keep a dear but obstinate father from leaving home, how to keep ourselves firmly in hand, and how to get some sleep. We don't need to look for other petty problems.

Long-Distance Caregiving

Nancy is the child of an Alzheimer's patient. She lives with her family in one state and worries about her aging parents in a state 800 miles away. What is happening to them on a day-to-day basis? The role of long-distance caregiver is very difficult:

> My mom and dad have been married for fifty-four years and are still deeply in love. Every time I talk to my dad he tells me how wonderful Mom is and what good care she takes of him. He calls her "The Big Magoo."
>
> I have no doubt that my mom is providing the best care she can for my dad. My concern is how much longer her care alone will be enough. I recently asked her if he'd seen his neurologist lately and she said, "Not for a year. There's really no point."
>
> My dad has congestive heart failure and is seen by a cardiologist, a hematologist, and an internist—but the three specialists don't communicate. When Dad was recently referred to a thoracic surgeon to discuss his lung tumor, Dad's cardiologist hadn't even told him about the Alzheimer's. When I spoke to the surgeon on the phone and mentioned it, he said, "Oh, that explains his lack of effect." *Duh!*
>
> My concern is that I don't really know what's going on. I'm in Dallas and they're in Kentucky. Last week, I came home in the evening and saw on my caller ID that Mom had called that morning but hadn't left a message. We had just spoken the day before. I called her back and asked her if anything was wrong and she said no, but sounded like she was trying not to cry. Of course, Dad was in the room and he gets upset when she's on the phone. So the only time she'd even consider talking openly is if he is napping. At night, if he goes to bed, he wants her to come too, even if it's 9:00 P.M. and she's not in the least tired.

It's nearly impossible for Nancy to know what is going on in her parents' home. Her mother needs support, and she is too far away to provide it, but she is emotionally close enough to her parents to see that her mother is beginning to show stress cracks. Her father doesn't want Mother on the phone, and the constant shadowing common to many Alzheimer's patients creates huge stress. One caregiver confided that her

Alzheimer's husband wouldn't even let her go to the bathroom alone. Under such circumstances, it won't be long before Nancy may have to care for both parents.

Several scenarios can evolve from this simple story. Mother can have a nervous breakdown or physical collapse. Father may have to be placed in an assisted-living facility or nursing home. Or Nancy could hire a case manager to check on her parents from time to time. Perhaps she could arrange some in-home respite care to allow her mother to have a peaceful shopping trip or library time. Her father might even be encouraged to attend a daycare facility a few days a week. Well, there it is! Now that I don't need the answers, I appear to know them all.

Not Everything Has An Answer

We've said it before, but it bears repeating: There just *are* times when there are no solutions. These are the days when we just have to sit in a corner and wait it out. My friend shares such a time:

> I've come to believe that we can live too long. My father-in-law is now in constant pain and is incontinent, but he has enough awareness to be embarrassed and humiliated by his infirmities. His doctor doesn't believe in painkillers, and this has caused me nothing but anguish as I watch him living in extreme pain day after day. He can no longer walk with a walker and must rely on someone else to get him around in a wheelchair. He hates his existence, and last night he cried himself to sleep. I cried right along with him. As we cried together, I cursed the medical establishment for allowing him to experience a life of relentless pain with no relief in sight. He is incredibly healthy due to modern medicine, but his life is hell. I fully understand a caregiver wanting to bring his loved one some peace from this kind of existence.
>
> I've just finished my third night with hardly any sleep as I listen for him trying to get out of bed. If he gets up and falls when I'm alone with him, I cannot pick him back up. I've had to call Fire Rescue once when my husband was gone after he fell while trying to go to the bathroom. I know the lack of sleep is causing me to become easily frustrated and angry.
>
> Last night my father-in-law managed to get himself into the hallway, transfer himself into the wheelchair, and then wedge himself

sideways between the walls in the hallway. He was wet but wouldn't allow me to change him. He insisted that he was not wet, and when I pointed to his soaked pajama bottoms he cried and still said he was not wet and didn't want to be changed. I have an aide who has agreed to stay every day until he is in bed. We have a urinal beside the bed. But, as others have mentioned, his reasoner is broken, and his pride will not allow him to let me help him.

I've taken him to the doctor twice in the last two weeks to find the source of his pain. The X-ray of his spine was negative for a fracture. The doctor says it is "just arthritis" and won't give him pain relief. I find it hard to believe that arthritis can appear so suddenly and cause such debilitating pain. I can't imagine myself enduring this misery twenty-four hours a day with no end in sight.

I'm tired and feeling more powerless than I ever have in my entire fifty-four years of life. I'm taking him back to the doctor today. I don't know what good it will do, but I've got to do something.

She speaks for so many of us. There just aren't any magic pills. If we look at the combination of stress factors here, it is amazing: lack of sleep, physical inability, mental stress, heartache for her father-in-law, and lack of communication with and support from the doctor. Add to this her father-in-law's lifetime modesty and desire to master his own fate, and the situation is unbearable for them both.

The compassion she feels for her father-in-law hurts almost as much as the actual job of caring for him. What really hurts is that there seems to be no way to help him. Two possible options might help the situation: get another doctor's opinion about pain medications and/or consider an assisted-living facility or a nursing home where trained staff can help him. As my friend says, "I've got to do something."

And then, suddenly, it all somehow seems to make sense. Ethelinn's family was chosen to be on a recent PBS documentary called "And Thou Shalt Honor." Yes, this program honors our Alzheimer's loved ones, but as Ethelinn says:

> . . . it also honors us . . . the caregivers. It makes me realize the exact reasons why I answer the same question 10,000 times a day, why I live in a fortress, and how I have to juggle my life and make plans in advance to do the simplest of things for myself. And I suppose . . . no, I don't suppose . . . I know that I am honored to do this

for my father . . . aren't we all . . . for our fathers, mothers, spouses, grandparents, etc. It is our honor. And in honoring them we are honoring ourselves too, for our compassion, goodness and empathy, and, of course, love. Okay, okay, I can still say that after my father has spit on the floor, pooped in the shower, and called his caregiver a prostitute—in Polish.

I wrote to Ethelinn saying:

> It isn't every family that can say they "honor their Alzheimer's loved one," so your letter made me think about honor. Whenever I want to investigate a word, I go back to the Latin I took in school. God knows why, but I did, and as it does many times, it helped me think about the word "honor" in a way I had never done before. The word "honos" in Latin means much as it does in English, but my Latin dictionary also mentioned the idea of sacrifice associated with honor. In honoring our elders or spouses, we provide a sacrifice toward both the person and the spiritual. My daughter reminded me that her yoga classes end with the phrase, "Namaste—I salute the divinity within you." Thus, by sacrificing for our loved one, we link them and ourselves to something beyond ourselves. True honor can only benefit the giver as well as the receiver.

And here is the *best* caregiving advice available:

> *And somehow I do cope, not well, but I do cope.*
> *Wanna know the secret?*
> *Ben and Jerry's Triple Caramel Chunk.*
> *. . . although there are days when maybe*
> *I just might hate that too!*
> —Ethelinn

SIX
A Few Extra Moments, Please

The Alzheimer's Association has a card that says it all. It can be handed to clerks or waiters when you take your loved one for an outing. It reads:

> *Thank you for your patience. The person with me is memory-impaired and may require a few extra moments. Your understanding is appreciated.*[1]

Patience, time, and understanding; it's not too much to ask, is it?

Grandma's Fairy Words

The loss of short-term memory is dreadful, but the loss of vocabulary is even worse. It is extremely difficult to understand the short-circuited language of Alzheimer's. One man did nothing but repeat his wife's name over and over, all day long. Another patient repeated "help" at the top of her lungs. In such cases understanding is of little help, but for many patients, conversation retains a wealth of meaning, if only the listener is able to fill in the missing gaps.

Rob and his wife, Didi, are very family oriented and were aware of Rob's mother's struggle to communicate. It is obvious that they put great effort into translating Alzheimer's Talk. Can we learn to read between the lines as they did?

The words Rob's mother used seemed to come from the poetic, silvery part of her self, and what a beautifully rich, encompassing self it was. Didi was wise enough to write down the seemingly meaningless mumblings and try to fill in the blanks. As a result, the family has a lasting memory of their mother and grandmother. I have included the original version of Grandma's Christmas message and Didi's translated version. It is a lesson in overcoming the communication barrier. Here is what Grandma *actually* said:

> It's a heck of a time to tell someone, but I'm not going to worry about it. Not presentation of your problem. We're trying to find a

half-lost. . . . are you aching to know? Just because I'm "sick" sort of on the edge of that and out of the freedom doesn't mean that I (don't) wish I could be with people that I care about a whole lot.

I'm so happy that you wanted to be home for Christmas. People are different in their ways, their clothing, their health. Sometimes, we can't be at the same place at the right time. When there are a lot of people around me it's like a "chorus piece." The house is falling down. Please don't have a "deaf attitude." Sometimes my words are paltry, and it bothers me. So listen to my *fairy words*, the color is six, and if you listen hard you can hear the sound on the water and the butterfly wings.

I've gotta tell you, you are query ducks. Can you hear yourselves, quack, quack, quack, why, why, why? I'm going to be all that I can be. When he (Dad) comes home, he just brightens up the whole room. White socks dirty up a little soon. Catch on to the concessions, depends on how easily we can sway. We have light phases and some low flying myrtle days. Have the strength, until the fire alarm. Be on top of that. Carnivorous animals. We have to cuddle up keepers of the light. We, ourselves, chant when our views are pure. Hounding sate the birds—private nights.

Your love points keep growing. You look happy. You stand up and look around. That's part of it. How can you think of anything except—"Wonderful"? Sometimes strict song. Teachers wear chocolate or be stone. We get spoiled easily and some of it is good and some of it is bad. And if you don't get what you want, just put it at the end of the line. We have jumbo features, pad your abilities and a real fever for it. Right away. Swimmer in the water, third basket to the right, second floor. Orndu Orndu, Dolger and Saushed.

Land petal happy, to sing and dance and have time to sit on the steps. Be spontaneous. Cloud searching. Dress warm, icicles on your dresses, Carley and Em. A bell rings true (when it doesn't) have an exaggerated sound. I didn't save enough time. . . . We need more time for Christmas. Well, as long as we have the decorations here, we can just go by. Maybe if we have some more presents. Is taking up someone else's cart. I think that comes out of our family. As long as you love that much, I'm sure everything will turn out just spoofy! We wanted to do so much good. We love you. We hope you have a great day.

What follows is Didi's interpretation of what Mom meant to say on Christmas Day:

"It's a heck of a time to tell someone, but I'm not going to worry about it." It's not always easy to make a "presentation of your problem. We're trying to find a half-lost . . . Are you aching to know?" Just because I'm "sick," sort of on the edge of that and out of the freedom, doesn't mean that I (don't) wish I could be with people that I care about a whole lot." I'm so happy that you "wanted to be home for Christmas. People are different in their ways, their clothing, their health." Sometimes, "we can't be at the same place at the right time." When there are a lot of people around me it's like a "Chorus piece." But sometimes it feels like the "house is falling down." Please don't have a "deaf attitude." Sometimes my words are "paltry, and it bothers me." So listen to "my fairy words, the color is six" and if you listen hard you can "hear the sound on the water and the butterfly wings."

"I've gotta tell you, you are query ducks." Can you hear yourselves, "Quack, quack, quack, why, why, why?" "I'm going to be all that I can be. When he (Dad) comes home, he just brightens up the whole room." We know "white socks dirty up a little soon. Catch on to the concessions," our good marriage "depends on how easily we can sway. We have light phases and some low flying myrtle days." We don't wait to "have the strength, until the fire alarm. Be on top of that." We're not just "carnivorous animals. We have to cuddle up." Be "keepers of the light. We, ourselves, chant when our views are pure. Hounding" each other doesn't help. Take time to "sate the birds." We enjoy our "private nights."

For my dear grandchildren: " Your love points keep growing. You look happy. You stand up and look around. That's part of it. How can you think of anything except "Wonderful"? Sometimes "it's necessary for your parents to sing you a "strict song. Teachers" can't always "wear chocolate or be stone. We get spoiled easily and some of it is good and some of it is bad. And if you don't get what you want, just put it at the end of the line. We have jumbo features," and you all have "padded your abilities." You all have special interests "and a real fever for it." You want it "right away." Eric, you're a super athlete, Carley and Emily you're super swimmers, Ben you're a super writer. "Swimmer in the water, third basket to the right, second floor." Ben, I'm glad you are writing about a planet named "Orndu, using my fairy words, Orndu, Dolger and Saushed."

We have a very special family. Sometimes I look at it as living on a "land petal." I want you children to be "happy, to sing and dance and have time to sit on the steps. Be spontaneous." Have fun "cloud searching. Dress warm." I don't want you to get "icicles on your dresses, Carley and Em. A bell rings true (when it doesn't) have an exaggerated sound. I didn't save enough time . . . We need more time for Christmas. Well, as long as we have the decorations here, we can just go by. Maybe if we have some more presents. Part of Christmas is taking up someone else's cart. I think that comes out of our family. As long as you love that much, I'm sure everything will turn out just spoofy! We wanted to do much good. We love you. We hope you have a great day."

I hope the reader can take the time to read over Grandma's fairy words once again. Enjoy the beautiful, poetic phrases (myrtle days) and literary statements (cuddle up to the keepers of the light). And I love one of her last sentences, "As long as you love that much, I'm sure everything will turn out just spoofy."

Making the effort to understand the Alzheimer's patient often brings delightful rewards. Consider the "spoofy" feelings we now have for Grandma after we understand her beautiful words and compare them to our feelings after reading the Alzheimer's version. First, we felt confusion and dismissed the speaker and the ideas, but when we took the time to listen and translate, we gained appreciation and respect for what she was trying to say.

Looking back, I wish my ears had been able to "hear" between the lines when Mother was ill. Alzheimer's speech becomes garbled, but the purity of soul sometimes shows between the lines. On occasion, if we teach ourselves to listen, Alzheimer's can show us what is left when all inhibitions and all structured, learned devices have been taken from us. Sometimes we can hear our loved one's soul singing in the void.

There are those magical times when Alzheimer's patients make points with startling clarity. It isn't always easy to listen between the lines. Sometimes we hear things we don't wish to hear. I recall Uncle W. who lived in Mother's Alzheimer's wing at her nursing home. Uncle W. could be quite a handful. He had been born in Europe and had had a very responsible position in one of our premier hotels. One day when I was visiting, Uncle W. stared at me for a moment and, obviously mistaking me for someone else, spoke in English for the first time in years. I will never forget his words. He shook his fist and said, "Look at you! You have everything, and I have nothing. Nothing!" I know now that he was, unfortunately, right.

The Depth of Alzheimer's

My first insight into the staggering mysteries of Alzheimer's occurred on the day we took our new grandchild into the Alzheimer's ward to meet his great-grandmother. She reached out to him with all the love and feeling of eternal motherhood. Hesitantly I handed him to her, ready to catch him should she fumble or forget. To my amazement all the ladies in the wing were suddenly surrounding us.

At this point I was an uneducated, rather fearful learner concerning Alzheimer's, and I felt a bit of panic. What if they grabbed at him? What if they screamed and scared him? What if they began fighting with one another? None of this happened. Instead, they all began coo-ing and "goochy-gooing" like normal grandmothers, stroking his small head and asking questions. "How old is he?" "Is it a boy?" "What's his name?" For a moment these frayed and broken lives were brought into focus. It didn't last long, but it was beautiful. At the emotional, instinc-tual level, for that moment, they were whole human beings.

We caregivers are often so aware of personal loss and painful emotions that we automatically take the depressing view that the loved one is lost to everything. This is far from true. In their excellent book, *The Best Friends Approach to Alzheimer's Care,* Virginia Bell and David Troxel list some of the common emotions that trouble the Alzheimer's person: loss, isolation and loneliness, sadness, confusion, worry and anxiety, frustra-tion, fear, paranoia, anger, and embarrassment. (12).

In *Coping With Alzheimer's,* Rose Oliver and Frances Bock agree:

> While losing her (the Alzheimer's patient's) cognitive abilities, she still maintains the ability to feel. She has emotions—some blunted, some exaggerated—but she can still feel anger, pain, sorrow, hurt, gladness, and pleasure. She can respond to affection, to approval, to an acknowledgement that she is a worthwhile person. She is strug-gling for affirmation of her humanity. (194).

This reminds me of Gladys, a fellow traveler with my mother. Gladys yearned to go home, more than any patient I had ever seen. She asked everyone that entered the wing to "please take me home." One day, a young man visiting in the unit responded to her plea with the self-conscious laugh of one unused to being around dementia. He meant no harm. Gladys turned and in her most school-teachery voice said, "Are you laughing at me?" Yes, they are still "in there." It just takes a bit of patience to find them. All right, agreed. At times it takes more than a little bit of patience.

Whit Garberson, a social worker in Boston, has worked extensively with the elderly and has a way of putting things so I can understand them:

> Dementia gurus point out what I think we all know intuitively: emotion is the last thing to go. Short-term memory, problem solving, judgment, concentration, insight, and all the other components of "executive function" may erode partially or completely, but the ability to experience emotion almost always persists.
>
> Add to this some of what researchers are saying about how memory works: experiences and learning seem to be stored in different ways depending on how much emotion and/or the importance of survival is associated with them.
>
> On the deepest and most hard-wired level of memory, the realm where a day-old chick runs from the shadow of a hawk but not the shadow of a pigeon, many of us react instinctively to snakes, fire, or the smell of decay.
>
> At the extreme opposite end of the scale—way up near the surface—we take in information all the time and then discard it because it has no emotional value: the name of someone met in passing, the address of a great website. Our brains are not designed to catalog hundreds of names and faces for quick retrieval.
>
> We retain a name if in some way, either positively or negatively, an experience touched us. I had a huge fear of spiders for decades until I saw *The Thief of Baghdad* a few years ago and realized I had seen it as a very young child and been terrified by the scene of the boy stuck in the giant spider's web. I nearly wet my pants when the scene came around, while my eight-year-old son sat there, a bit bored by the lousy special effects, wondering what the big deal was. For me, that memory was down quite deep.
>
> I imagine a sort of RAM area in the brain, a buffer system that largely gets deleted every night when the machine is turned off, unless a piece of data is associated with strong affect or survival, in which case it gets written to disk. I imagine there are parts of the

disk that are more secure than others against erasure, perhaps depending on how often we access them.

As I see it, all of this helps explain why it is possible to work with demented folks if we focus on speaking to their feelings and de-emphasize the factual. It helps explain why, when somebody puts on her best clothes and sets off down the nursing home corridor announcing she is going to meet her long-dead father at the dock and sail to Europe, it is not helpful to say, "Now Barbara, you live here now, and your father died fifty years ago." I find this is a surprisingly tough point to make to certain nurses who apparently have been trained to think that "redirection" and "reorientation" are more important than empathic connection. What about "You've been missing your father?" or "Let me walk with you. Now tell me about him, will you?"

Naomi Feil, a social worker from the Cleveland area and author of *Validation Breakthrough*, can be credited with many of the techniques recommended today. Ms. Feil has taught her communication techniques throughout the world, and they have been adopted in some of the most forward-thinking facilities for demented patients from Germany to Kansas. Major points of her plan are:

1. Accept the person as they are today.
2. Understand that all communication has meaning, even if we don't understand it.
3. Understand that the meaning of the message lies under the direct statement.
4. A good way to get to the underlying message is to use reminiscence and props, including music, objects, pictures, and ourselves.
5. Get the person to discuss what they have just said. "Are you thinking of your mother right now?"
6. Wherever the patient is right now is good enough.
7. It pays to have a sense of humor.
8. Validation is a kinder approach than truth, reason, and trying to "retrain." It gives the patient a feeling of being accepted (Feil).

There are those who disagree in one way or another with this approach and sometimes caregivers are upset at those who would use "the therapeutic lie" with their loved ones. Raised to be honest people, it disturbs them to lie to a parent or spouse. When an eighty-five-year-old man is crying for his mother, however, is it best to say, "She's dead," a fact he will not retain, or is it best to distract him, to ask what she was like. In short, we can sympathize, empathize, pity, and pontificate. We can rationalize, yell, cry, grieve, and stress out to no avail. A simple look at the humanity of our loved one, listening to the emotions that lie there—somewhere beneath the surface—is our best path to understanding. It just takes a little patience.

A Fine Aloofness

Sometimes, through lack of concern or knowledge, family members or close friends just don't want to be bothered. It is a depressing characteristic of the disease that friends and relatives are in short supply when there is visiting to be done and even shorter supply when there is work to be done.

Mary laments the effect this has had on her husband:

> Gene, my husband, watches the driveway waiting for his old friends, anybody, to visit. Few people stop by. I don't know if they are embarrassed or have trouble talking to him. But it is sad. He used to have so many friends and now he imagines that he sees them driving down the road. I just can't get this across to them. Such is life.

Another spouse is aware of the same sad loneliness:

> I sent a Christmas letter explaining about my husband's illness and asked that people visit for a short period of time, just call and let me know when. He is German-born and now speaks mostly German. I thought he would enjoy visits from his old German friends. Well, no one has come and no one has called. His daughter lives about ten miles away and even she has not come. The last time she saw her dad was Thanksgiving two years ago. There will not be a funeral service. I do not want to hear the relatives and friends who could not spare a few hours telling me what a wonderful man he was and how much they will miss him.

That *poor man* we all speak of. That tragic scene we all decry. Unwilling to look honestly at what Alzheimer's is and unwilling to take the time to successfully deal with it, we practice a fine aloofness, a reluctance to engage in any direct grappling with its reality. We really don't want to know what is going on, and we sooth ourselves with *distancing words*, elbowing our demented friends into the far reaches of our retrieval system.

Do these refrains sound familiar?

- "She won't remember whether I was there so why go."
- "If he needs me, they'll let me know."
- "I don't want to be a bother."
- "If only they would place her in a home that's closer to us."
- "I don't think Aunt B. is as bad as they're saying. She's just getting old."
- "I always puddle up and cry, so I just don't go."
- "I want to remember him the way he was."
- "I just don't know what to say."
- "If that's what the future holds, I don't want to see it."
- "I'm just so darn busy!"

I am as guilty as anyone of using these pretexts. Expressions of self-protecting mechanisms, they keep reality and the demands of others from getting too close to our soft underbelly. Most of Mother's friends never bothered to visit, and all but one of those who did visit did so only once or twice. Isabel, our kind, long-time neighbor, was the exception. Armed with a bag of lemon drops or some other small token, she was the only friend brave enough to visit regularly. No one from Mother's church, which she had attended faithfully, ever came to our home to see her, and only the pastor went to see her once she was in the nursing home. They were unwilling to witness the living death of Elma. Either they attached no importance to being with her at this stage of her life, or they believed that once she didn't recognize them, it was no longer important. It didn't occur to them that they might give another human being a happy moment, regardless of her memory. They didn't see her standing at the window, looking into the distance, terribly alone in her disappearing mind. I made many mistakes in my caregiving, but my return journey has shown me where we all are guilty of neglect.

Pam has experienced the caregiver role at two levels and shares a different perspective with us. First she and her husband were caregivers at a distance, then for four years in which her mother lived with them in their home, and then in a nursing home. She reminds us to be a bit understanding of human error and to learn to ask for help:

I understand the problems of a caretaker after living it for a while now. A few years ago Mom cared for my dad for several years, as did my mother-in-law for her husband. We were caretakers from a distance then. There was a vast difference in our level of care at those times. I think a large part of it was ignorance. I don't think you can truly understand caretaker weariness and stress unless you have been one. I think that is one of the benefits of a support group. . . . My husband and I thought we did a good job helping our moms, but about all we did was visit and call. We tried to be supportive. We did what they asked but that was little. I don't think it was lack of care as much as lack of an understanding of what they were going through.

After Mom moved here and we were her full time caretakers, we understand what our moms had gone through caring for our dads. They never let us fully know of the stress and we didn't see it. Were we busy? Yes. Did we think we were helping? Yes. Were we of much help? Probably not. Would we have helped if we fully understood? Yes.

Those of us who have learned to live with this misunderstood disease, occasionally finding some pleasure in its elusive moments, know that as we accept the inevitable, we learn to cherish each moment and store away the memories of our departing loved one. If we refuse to give pleasure unless it will be remembered, if we are unable to access our humanity, then our focus is not on the person being pleased but on ourselves. The payback is unimportant. It doesn't matter if my loved one remembers. I will. It just requires a little patience and a great deal of empathy and understanding.

Stigma

"Have you noticed any reaction among your friends and acquaintances when you tell them that your mother is demented?" a friend asked. "Is it different than if you announced the onset of cancer? Is there a difference in the reaction?" "Stigma" is defined as "A mark . . . of infamy, disgrace, or reproach . . . a mark indicative . . . of a disease or abnormality." I did notice a difference in the reactions of some friends to Mother's illness, but I attributed it more to inexperience with the disease rather than an assumption of disgrace. I will admit that I sometimes try especially hard to remember names and dates when conversing with someone who knows Mother died with Alzheimer's. I worry that they may be thinking, "Oh, oh, I bet Sue's getting Alzheimer's." However, I assume the blame for this reaction. It is my own sense of the "stigma," the fear of inheriting this disease that inhibits me. What to the average person passes unnoticed, to someone afraid of inheriting Alzheimer's, a slight suggestion of inadequacy causes fear. My husband said today, "Boy! You've got a brain like a sieve!" It was said with love and humor, but it stopped me for a moment. Did I?

We have in the past "hidden" our demented relatives. We have been a mask for them, inventing excuses for their behavior and generally creating a culture of "no talk, hands off" when it comes to dementia. For so many years, dementia was not discussed, even among close family members. It will take a while before we will be willing to confide openly in our friends and relatives. The shame is not in the disease, however, but in the fact that we find it difficult to discuss openly.

Even today, families, not realizing they are ashamed, hesitate to tell friends and family of their loved one's affliction. When we could be getting support from those around us, we often pretend and cover and shut ourselves off from needed communication. Families are even afraid of having genetic tests done because of the danger that insurance companies or employers will learn of a possible inherited connection. This is understandable, and attitudes toward dementia will take a long time to change. The sad result is a culture virtually ignorant about how to deal with dementia and the demented.

After my mother was placed in an Alzheimer's unit, a good friend visited and promptly called me to task on the phone. "Can't you find a better place for your mother?" she fretted. "She just doesn't belong with *those people.*" Unprepared for a visit in the unpredictable environment of an Alzheimer's ward, she had fallen completely apart at the reality. She never visited my mother again. It takes a little patience and a lot of understanding.

I can appreciate this. I had the same reaction the first time I entered an Alzheimer's unit. I was honestly a bit afraid of these poor souls. Why? I think the unpredictability of each situation frightened me. God knows we all want to be in control, and control just isn't easily found in an Alzheimer's unit. Another problem for casual visitors is how to chat with a demented person. What do you say? With experience we develop some expertise, but at first it can be daunting. Nevertheless, with a little practice, one can enter a ward, hug Sally, shake hands with Bill, answer Grace's question about going home kindly saying, "Sorry, I can't take you home today. My car's broken." It just takes a little patience and understanding.

This is a skill I learned from a man named Bob, for whom I have the deepest respect. There was no stigma with Bob. Alzheimer's didn't prevent him from being comradely with these Alzheimer's patients. The minister of a small, local church, he visited Mother's unit every afternoon for about an hour. All of the residents recognized him, and he hugged and called each one by name, answering his or her endless questions with the patience of a saint. One day I walked to the car with him and told him how much I admired his loyalty to this group of twenty demented persons. His answer: "This is where it's at. Every theological student should have to spend one or two years in an Alzheimer's ward. Here you really see the human spirit." This should also apply to medical personnel in training, in my opinion.

After we have made our return journey, maybe that part of our overall task is to learn these skills and also give others a chance to learn. Our society is paying for hiding our demented and confused old folks, leaving barriers of misinformation that must be cracked. One friend made it a point to take his Alzheimer's wife out to dinner as often as possible. They enjoyed it, and the waitresses and frequent customers grew used to seeing them and developed a good relationship with his wife. Just as with the physically handicapped, society must be expected to make room for our Alzheimer's loved ones. Hospitals must improve their ability to deal with demented patients. Those who joke about dementia need education, and those with little patience need to practice that virtue. Looking back, I learned so much from my contact with Alzheimer's.

We tend to think of the rational as a higher order,
but it is the emotional that marks our lives.
One can often learn more from ten days of agony
than from ten years of contentment."
—Artist Helen Dudar

SEVEN
Tales of Laughter and Love

Peter sets us straight. Just when I start to feel a pity party coming on, I read something that Peter wrote, and I feel my emotional gyroscope beginning to steady:

> I agree, it is a horrible disease, but as hard as it may sound or seem, we can find rewards from our caring and compassion. We all get caught up in the feeling of helplessness, but another way to look at it is realizing they cannot change but that we can change in our way of looking and dealing with our loved ones. We can help them live in their highest–functioning ability. We can help them keep their self-esteem and dignity.
>
> One must look beyond the disease and try to touch those parts of their heart and soul, those moments of calm, the joys of a hug, the pleasure of a laugh. If we can change our way of looking at the disease and our loved ones, we can begin to enjoy the small joys along with some of the sorrows.

Or, as Lord Byron put it, "Adversity is the first path to Truth."

Harvard University's Herbert Benson, Duke University's Harold G. Koenig, and many others are currently exploring the connection between mind, spirit, and medicine. In his book *Timeless Healing: The Power and Biology of Belief,* Benson describes self-care, which includes cultivation of patients' inner resources to assist in their own healing as "the most disparaged and neglected aspect of health care today." He might add the neglected aspect of caregivers' health care to that statement.

Dr. Christina Puchalski, director of the George Washington University Institute for Spirituality and Health, is committed to the idea that "spirituality is a key dimension for achieving optimal health and for coping with illness." She defines spirituality as "that which allows a person to experience transcendent meaning in life. . . . Whatever beliefs and values give a person a sense of meaning and purpose in life" (Levathes, P HE01).

Attitude is all. Well, maybe not all, but it certainly affects reality. When I remember those caregiving years, I see them through a smaller viewfinder. It's as though my vision closed in during those Alzheimer's years, somewhat as it does with a migraine, and I was unable to see the truth, or in some cases, the best course of action. In fact, I think the experience colored all of my activities, causing me to react without humor, without foresight, and with a very negative and myopic outlook. I was a terrible grinch, but I blame the disease. It can make a grinch out of anyone.

The recently released report, *The Nuns' Study,* suggests that an optimistic, curious outlook on life led to the clarity and longevity in the lives of some nuns. The ability to view adversity with eyes sensitive to life's beauty and a mind capable of intercepting truth helps make life so dear. Caregivers who can look at the happenings of the moment and find meaning, humor, or love in those moments are blessed. Perhaps one day these memories will warm our hearts and ease our anger at this terrible disease.

This caregiver has found that the Alzheimer's experience has made her more aware of her connection to all living things:

> I remember my father trying to help a puppy that was hit by a car. The poor thing bit him. Instead of being angry at the puppy, he said it wasn't the dog's fault. It was in so much pain. I feel like that sometimes—filled with so much pain that I don't recognize a kind hand.

This is a moment to long remember from Carrie, whose husband has Alzheimer's:

> After lunch my loved one and I went to the grocery store. I left John (her Alzheimer's husband) in the car to listen to the music on the radio and to snooze—the first time I had done so. As I rounded an aisle in the store, there he was. He'd had to go to the bathroom. Of course the keys were locked in the car with the radio playing. AAA could not come for at least an hour, and I had a post-surgery occupational therapy appointment in fifteen minutes. So we took a

taxi to the occupational therapist, lugging two bags of groceries with us, and left sixty pounds of cat litter in the cart in front of the store.

Then back to the store by taxi with the groceries to find AAA just about to leave the parking lot. Happy ending: the battery was not dead, AAA got us into the car in a jiffy, the groceries did not spoil, and no one stole our kitty litter. Poor John, though. I told him he had better stay out of my way for a while. What a day. What a demonstration of how completely unpredictable this disease is.

C. shares a moment with her Alzheimer's mother:

I love to see the smile in Mum's eyes when she looks up at me. Minutes later the veil has fallen, but those few seconds are gold.

Beverly's story is one of my favorites:

Mother loves her little dog so much. She fed him jellybeans and everything else that she could find. When I repeatedly told her not to feed him, she would get angry with me and say, "Well, the kid's got to eat." I tried to explain that he was a dog and that would make her even more angry. With undeniably good logic, she would ask why I was letting her eat something that the dog should not have. I finally came up with the allergic story. It helped for about three seconds.

One day she informed me that she knew all about Bandit because she gave birth to him. I almost lost it. Now my mother is in a nursing home, and poor little Bandit is lost. No friend and no jellybeans, no love.

One thing Beverly's mother knew: the kid loved her, or at least he loved the jellybeans.

Here is another love story:

When his disease was about at stage six, my dad used to eat Oreos by the barrel-full. He would always have the telltale chocolate in the corners of his mouth. When he was doing all his night wanderings, he would come into my room. I would try—lovingly, strongly, and then finally like a bully—to get him back to bed, anything to get some sleep.

He would sometimes come in with Oreos and ask, "Do you want a cookie?" In my need for sleep, I would tell him it was the middle of the night. "Please get back to bed." One night, I was so worn out that I just took the cookie. Dad left and returned to bed all by himself. I was shocked. That night I received two more cookie deliveries. When my son came over the next morning, he kidded me about eating cookies in bed. I told him how I had received the cookies, and we had a big laugh together.

Looking back, however, I now realize that Dad was delivering love to me. Whenever I see a package of Oreos, I remember his nightly wanderings and miss getting his love. I loved him so much. The greatest tribute he ever paid me was about three months prior to his death. He introduced me as "Beverly, my wife and daughter." That seemed to mean that I met his needs.

Randy also found a moment to value:

I have found that finding humor in an otherwise really sad situation helps tons. My mom and dad have been married for fifty-one years. They still live together at home. At least half the time Dad thinks that Mom is just a woman who takes care of him at a care facility. This is noticeably taking its toll on Mom.

Sometimes, though, we all get a good laugh. For instance, Jan and I invited them for dinner to celebrate Father's Day. Before they came over, Dad told my mom that he and his wife were going to his son's house for dinner. Then he said, "I guess you're going to come, too. How do you think that will look?"

Funny? Maybe not to most people, but it certainly helped lighten the situation for all of us.

Then there are times that are funny but set the tears flowing. A caregiver shares one such moment with us:

This morning, when I made my trip to town to help Mother-in-law with her medication-taking, I said, "Well, you're up early, had your breakfast, and cleaned up the table. Lookin' bright-eyed and bushy-tailed. You're doing great this morning."

"Yes, well . . . " she replied, "Except I don't know where I am."

Cindi shares the story of Gremlin:

My mom, who lives with us, will be ninety in April and had a small red Doxie whom she loved a lot. It was funny. She can't remember my name or how we are related, but she always knew Gremlin.

I guess I was a little jealous. Well, poor little guy had to be put to sleep last Friday. Mother asks thirty times a day if we have seen him and gets up in the middle of the night to look for him. This has hit her hard. When she didn't feel like eating, Gremlin always got a goodie. We would sit outside the bathroom and wait for her. He did love her a lot. We were looking for another dog for her, but I don't know if she will accept the fact that Gremlin isn't coming back.

He slept in her room, and she worries that he doesn't have his blanket. She frets that he might have run away or is lost and cold. We remind her that he was very old, and now he is at peace.

After a few days of this and staying up until 4:30 with her, I decided it was time to check on another small dog. Yesterday, we went with her to the animal shelter and found a little Queensland Healer mix that had been a stray. Tuesday night we can bring her home, and Mom is counting the days until Tuesday. Last night she still asked for Gremlin. Strange, in her world of forgetfulness, Gremlin will not soon be forgotten.

In this world of forgetfulness, certain things take on exaggerated importance. Animals, children, music, and art—all are usually accepted and loved by Alzheimer's patients. Perhaps they represent the closeness, the innocence and gaiety, the beauty that makes life so dear. No, our loved ones haven't lost it all—at least not all of the important things of life.

And then there are memories that will be with us always. Helena has a home in the woods and happily raises her goats and tends her acres. A few years ago, her Alzheimer's mother came to live with her. I think her story has touched me the most for I know what happened later:

Mother and I collected our tree yesterday. I have a Christmas tree patch back up in the woods and it's certainly a trek to get there, mostly uphill on rough terrain, and I told Mother I was afraid she couldn't manage it. It was just too steep. "Hah," she said. And DID.

I'm astounded. An almost ninety-four-year-old lady who's so frail generally that I even hesitate taking her to the mall for shopping, managed this three-fourth-mile trek uphill. Not only did she manage it, but after I'd cut the tree, plus one more for greenery and goat nibbling, she also hauled the greenery on back *down* the hill. Granted these are slim trees, treelings really, but ain't life amazing.

She didn't hear the turkeys, however. They were settling into the trees for the night and were full of bedtime chatter, and I loved hearing them. As I told her, I've wanted to share my Christmas with her for sixteen years, and I am simply overjoyed to finally have her here. She wept happy tears. So did I.

Ho! Ho! Ho!

Not long afterwards, Helena's mother was diagnosed with pancreatic cancer. She lived only a few more months. With the same tender care she gave her animals, Helena watched over her mother's final days and savored the last moments of her life, knowing she would find truth and beauty in the experience. Well done.

Carolyn has another memory to cherish:

> Mom, stage five or six and unable to finish a sentence, had been in the assisted-living facility for months and had adjusted well. The period before moving to the AFL was traumatic to say the least. There were weeks in a psychiatric hospital to get her medications adjusted and a few weeks in a rehabilitation facility.
>
> I was visiting Mom when a new Alzheimer's neighbor came out of her room. I said hello to this new person as we walked toward the elevator to go for a walk. The neighbor announced very loudly that she had a son who lived in town and another son who lived nearby, but that *she* lived in Chicago. Mom, with a knowing look, said, "Not anymore, you don't."

One wonders just how demented Uncle Raymond was in this story from Geri. Who will ever forget Uncle Raymond?

> Uncle Raymond would go into a particular restaurant and insist he was going to have "the special: three pancakes and the salad bar, and I'm only paying $3.65." The waiters would patiently, then impatiently, try to tell him that that special had ended several years ago. Well, old Ray was dumb like a fox. First he would get loud. Then he would bang the table with his fist, saying, "I'm going to

have THREE PANCAKES AND THE SALAD BAR, AND I'M ONLY GOING TO PAY THREE DOLLARS AND SIXTY-FIVE CENTS . . . "

Dan and I wanted to crawl under the table. But you know what? He always got THREE PANCAKES AND THE SALAD BAR, AND HE ONLY PAID THREE DOLLARS AND SIXTY-FIVE CENTS. Now, whenever Dan and I go into a fancy restaurant, one of us always says, "I WANT . . ."

Janine's mother, age eighty-five, has always been a flirt, but dementia has removed all her inhibitions about saying what she really thinks:

We were in the eye doctor's office and he asked her to read the letters on the chart. She looked at him and said, "I'd rather look at you." He promptly blushed. This happened not once, but twice, and on the third visit to the optician, the nurse gave the eye chart test. I must add that Mother has good taste, as he is a very good looking man.

And we can't forget Ethelinn's father—you know, the one who wanted to go home to L.A.:

My father was watching a Marx Brothers movie and could not remember their names. I kept telling him, but of course he kept forgetting them. Finally, after so many times of this, he came into the kitchen very proudly telling me that he can remember the names of the Marx brothers: Harpo, Chico . . . and Karl.

And then we remember the professional caregivers. As Peter said, some are wonderful and some not so. We also discover that there are all kinds. Carla describes one she'll never forget:

There was a wonderful physical therapist who did rehab work with my mother in the nursing home. This woman had a heavy German accent. She was a taskmaster and accepted no excuses or malingering, letting my mother's abuse and curses roll right off her back. "Yes, yes I am . . . and now ve take another step, see . . . " I fell in love with her; she didn't take the least bit of abuse from my mother, and she got her mobile. But when she discovered the first day that my mother was wearing a gown and no underwear under it, she spun around and said to me, "Und VERE are her PANTS?" I said, "In her room; she won't put them on." She whirled back to my mother and snapped, "In ZIS hospital VE VEAR ze UNDER-PANTS." Mother wore them every day after that.

Peter, once again, brings us back from our chuckles and laughter to other memories equally as warm and thoughtful:

> The Holiday Hospice Ceremonies, with their spirit of remembrance, loss, and memoriam; the Light a Light program, with the lights on the trees in Boston Common reminding us of those we have loved and lost—this is the spirit of community, which allows me to deal with that dark place.
>
> For me this is the soul of holiday memories of loss, closure. It is extremely personal but also done in a community so we are not alone. I liked to have dinner at the nursing home with Mother that night and be left alone. No false sense of obligation and surrounded by people who will let me be.

And so we laugh and so we cry, finding comfort where we can: a chuckle here, a tear there, looking around the shadows into something precious that we can only glimpse and do not yet understand. Perhaps, like our Alzheimer's loved ones, we too are looking for home.

> *Only that day dawns to which we are awake.*
> *There is more day to dawn.*
> *The sun is but a morning star.*
> —Henry David Thoreau

Alzheimer's can be the pathway on which we glimpse something more than that which is. It is a great "aha" disease. By living through this disease with a loved one, we see a glimpse of the morning star—just a glimpse. Angels are often present in the writings of Alzheimer's caregivers and even in the artwork of patients far advanced in the disease. One of the most lovely and yet most primitive pictures of "Spirit" was painted by an Alzheimer's patient shortly before her death. Given watercolors and paper, she shaped what could only be described as a pink angel, round, comforting, and thought-provoking.

The vulnerability that Alzheimer's brings may help us see the hidden love, beauty, and humor in our lives. We suddenly begin to cherish the small things in life, for sometimes that is all we have. Just as blindness leads the unsighted to a greater use of the other senses, so Alzheimer's, which blocks the normal pathways of the brain, leads our loved ones to unforeseen insights. If we're lucky, they will, perhaps, enrich us, too. At the very least, they may leave us with some wonderful memories of laughter and love, those things that make life rich and full.

EIGHT
Guilty Decisions

*These are days when no one should
rely unduly on his "competence."
Strength lies in improvisation. All the
decisive blows are struck left-handed.*

—Walter Benjamin

When Alzheimer's first strikes, we have the tendency to put off making
any decision because we are afraid of making the wrong decision. We
engage in a frantic search for control. If we do make a decision, we
question it over and over. "Should I have done that?" "Maybe we should
have done this." "What doctor? What Medicine? What! No medicine.
Oh, dear. What next?" Perhaps that is why I hesitated to ask advice: I
didn't want anyone to see just how inept I was, using silly reasoning and
a typical protectionist attitude.

Actually, in Alzheimer's, many of our best blows, though awkward,
are struck left-handed. Creative solutions, sometimes stopgap in nature,
are often best. Few decisions made in Alzheimer's care are permanently
successful. What works today may not be successful tomorrow. The best
caregivers are loose, relaxed, and able to flow with the tide. Take, for example, Ethelinn. She decided to take her father's shoes away to keep
him from wandering. If it works, it's a good decision. If it doesn't, she
will have to try something else. The controlled personality might make
the same decision and then become stressed and upset if the strategy
failed.

Creative solutions, however, are hard for many to make. We can give
lip service to "living in our loved one's reality," but try to do it. Few of
us have the patience Carlene showed with her father:

It has made life so much easier. Once I was able to enter his reality, my father stopped having catastrophic reactions and seemed to settle down. Granted, this is not easy to do, but once you can master it, your life will be so much easier for you and your loved one.

My family and I all enter his world and he seems to be much happier since we have been able to do this. We sit in the car with him driving and go on rides (even though we never leave the driveway). I let him wear my Birkenstocks and I wear his cowboy boots. I have helped him mix dog food and bird seed and then spread it on the garage floor. I have taken him to the store with him wearing two hats. We have moved furniture, and I have had a wheelbarrow full of firewood in MY bedroom. I could go on for hours about the strange things that go on in this house. I have people tell me that I am "indulging" my father too much. As long as he seems happy and what we are doing is not harmful, I do whatever he wants. It does take a lot of extra time to clean up things and rearrange furniture once he's in bed, but his calmness and happiness are worth the extra work it may cause me. "Okay, Dad, whatever you say, Dad," is something that I must say fifteen times a day.

As a caregiver, I picture myself flailing away at the disease, sword in both hands. Instead of creatively taking a left-handed slash at our problems, I hacked away awkwardly and only slightly wounded the disease that was stealing my mother from me and trying unsuccessfully to keep everything "rational." We know that Alzheimer's will win and that no decision we make is permanently helpful. Sometimes no choices are available, and sometimes we are confounded if we do and confounded if we don't.

If we want to beat ourselves up for the mistakes made in caring for our loved one, there is an endless array of weapons at our disposal. We can insist that we should have placed her in a different assisted-living facility or chosen another medication or tried to make him happier. We can demand qualities of ourselves that only angels possess. Good caregivers are the hardest on themselves, but I must admit, I now realize that no matter how perfect I tried to be, sadly, *I made no good decisions during Mother's illness. I just made the best I could at the moment.*

Several years later, I reflect on one decision that still triggers great feelings of guilt. It was a quiet July morning when, full of pain, I led

Mother out of her home for the last time—the *last* time. True, it was the best decision, but not a good decision. If I had had more information or more money, I might have made a better decision, but at the time I didn't see any alternatives. I still shudder when I think of the finality of it all, and I wish I had had a better option. Poor dear soul, she didn't deserve to be deprived of her home and treasures and to be forced to spend her last years among strangers. On the other hand, when placed in capable hands, she became busy, active, involved in a community, and safe. So, it was not a good decision, but it was the best decision I could make at the time. And I learned from this experience. I learned that there are wonderful, caring strangers out there who know more about most things than I do. I learned to trust.

When death beckoned Mother and twentieth-century medicine was at my disposal to help her live just a little longer, I had to make the best decisions I could. But they weren't good decisions. It is never good to withhold added time from a human life, but we make life and death choices based on the facts as we know them. We remove loved ones from a beloved home, we place them in small rooms in our homes or in institutional settings we usually don't even want to visit, and we limit medications and treatment in final moments. These are not good decisions, but they're the best we know how to make at this place and time.

How can one decide between hell and hell? Those seemed to be my only choices. We choose, unhappily, because we must, living with our decisions as best we can, returning to reconsider them again and again, chewing them over like a dog with a bone. Did I pick the right path? Would it have been better had I chosen this alternative or that? Resignation and acceptance, not certitude and never peace, are the only finale for the carer. I am sure there are souls on this earth who can make such decisions cavalierly, without a thought to the outcome. I am not one of them. To me, I only feel comfortable making personal choices for myself, not for others.

I have met only one caregiver who really seemed to enjoy having control over the life of his Alzheimer's spouse. It was a bit like having his own Barbie doll. He told her when to eat, what to eat, and where to sit; he arranged all clothing choices and diaper changes with the skill and composure of a top sergeant. Most of us aren't like this. The decisions we are forced to make for someone else drain our emotional reserves. We feel intrusive and meddlesome, but "somebody's gotta do it."

Do what? Decide what? Just about everything. In most other illnesses, the patient can retain his decision-making ability until well along in the disease. Unfortunately, even in the early stages of Alzheimer's, the family will have to make tough decisions. When should she take her medicines and how can that be arranged now that she can't remember to do so? We have to decide when she should see a doctor and what kind of doctor. Does she need dental care? What can I do when she doesn't want to bathe or change her clothes? How can I protect her when she begins to wander? Is she safe at home? Unlike toddlers who can be put in a playpen, eighty-year-olds are not so easy to protect. Safety becomes a major problem. Keeping them from eating things that will harm them, burning down the house, or wandering away forever become mind-consuming projects. Is it safe for him to sit in the car while I shop? How can we stop him from driving?

Caregivers spend much of their time wondering which dead bolt or cabinet lock will keep father home or prevent him from stripping in the middle of the mall. We scope medical supply catalogs with all the concentration once devoted to CD choices. What is the best alarm device? Has anyone tried that style of Depends? Hmmmm. We fuss, we stew, we decide.

But then come many more difficult decisions. What do we do if our loved one refuses to accept the fact that she can no longer live alone? How can we force her to get a doctor's diagnosis if she chooses not to? Which doctor should I take her to? What medications should my loved one take? Can you arrange your home so that she can live with you? Should we move in with her? Can I give up my life to care for her?

Our minds whirl with the disorder. However, we do have another option. We can choose not to choose. We can just let it happen. What if he insists on climbing stairs and driving cars when he is no longer able? Am I going to let him? As the condition worsens, we worry that he should not be alone at all. Rotten food collects in her refrigerator; the neighbors have to return her to her home more and more often. She has had one accident in the car, and she has fallen once. We can say, "Well, it was only once," and blame our indecision on "Mom doesn't want to move." Or we can make decisions—not good ones, not ones she's going to like—based on her safety. At a certain stage in Alzheimer's, we often cannot make our loved ones happy, we can only keep them safe. Then we have to decide: home aides, day care, assisted living, nursing home, move her in with us? Anybody have any good ideas? And this is not the time to flip a coin.

If you have a durable power of attorney (DPOA), usable even if the person is demented, you can literally, in most situations, decide between life and death. That's an oversimplification, but in most states the DPOA can arrange for DNR (Do Not Resuscitate) orders and can sign the papers necessary for nursing home placement, surgery, and the use or nonuse of medical procedures such as tube feeding and even administration of antibiotics.

Judith Klein, a psychotherapist-caregiver in N.Y.C engaged in treating caregivers with similar problems, kindly shares her personal experience with us:

> How much should we honor a loved one's wish to die rather than experience the later stages? And how much do other family's wishes count? These are Solomon-like decisions that we faced two years ago.
>
> My mother, then eighty-five and in stage three or four, suddenly stopped eating after a stomach virus. With her electrolyte balance thrown off, her blood pressure dropped precipitously; she collapsed and was hospitalized. They stabilized her by feeding her through an I.V. Once off the I.V. she still refused to eat, and the doctors recommended a feeding tube, which we were all in agreement we didn't want. They were then prepared to send her home to die. All this changed when we convinced the doctors that we thought she was depressed and we had her transferred to a psych unit. Once the antidepressants kicked in she began to eat again. We took this move because my father was not ready to lose her and especially I don't think he could have tolerated taking her home and watching her die by starvation.
>
> Fast forward the tape two years and Mother is now near the end of the sixth stage and in a nursing home. We have been through endless crises and she is in a very deteriorated state. (She speaks, eats, walks, smiles very little, is aggressive periodically, and doesn't know family except my father.) I wonder now if I made the right choice.

I think Mother's intent was to die two years ago, but I was caught between what both my parents needed. They needed different things, and my father could advocate for what he needed.

I feel guilty at times for "saving her life." Saved for what? Misery. It now seems like a cruel choice. I think it takes a great deal of soul searching to make the right choice.

Caregivers often say, "I don't want to think about that time." Who does? But the decisions are there whether one likes it or not. Caregivers who have gone this far say it's better to consider these questions ahead of time. As the above caregiver says, "It requires serious soul searching."

Mother lapsed into a coma the last week of her life and I, being an only child, had to decide whether to give her IV feedings. I was told the day before she died that she had a major infection. What to do? "Do you want to give her antibiotics?" the doctor's assistant asked. We opted for the antibiotics but did not offer an I.V. feeding. I do not regret this choice. Mother had nothing to come back to, but I just regret having to make such a decision.

At the risk of making it more difficult for the caregiver than it already is, we have to remind ourselves that each case, each person, each family is different, and only the family can make these choices. Guilt accompanies almost every decision. Placing a loved one in an institutional setting, or even a boarding home, invites plenty of guilt. I still have dreams, five years after Mother died, that she suddenly becomes well enough to bring home. I call this my "Alice in Wonderland Dream," but then I awaken. Reality speaks and I know that all the decisions I had to make were due to one fact: Alzheimer's is progressive. We have to adjust our decisions to it, it does not adjust to us.

A good friend made a very scary decision to leave his aging father at home under dangerous circumstances, until finally the father, after several frightening episodes, *asked* to go to a care facility. Ironically, he fell soon after arriving at the nursing home, broke his hip, and died from the results of surgery. So, what was the best decision?

I sometimes think that whatever I say or do to my grown children will be the wrong thing: If I question, I'm prying; if I give suggestions, I'm criticizing; if I do nothing, I don't care. Caregivers are caught in the same muddle, damned if we do and damned if we don't. Family members, absent from the day-to-day care, inevitably will criticize what the caregiver does, and friends purse lips at your choices. I used to believe I was at the bottom of a snake pit with Mother and neither one of us could get out. Sadly, as an only child, I had no siblings that could help me deal with the decisions of this awful tragedy; part of my feelings of aloneness were my own fault. I shut out a lot of help.

Recent research shows that a frightening number of caregivers die before the Alzheimer's loved one passes on. Caregiving is a physically-demanding, sleep-depriving, mentally-exhausting job, and the decisions we have to make cause unmitigated stress. So be careful. For me, the guilt and lack of confidence in my caregiving decisions hurt the most. J. has found peace with one difficult decision, but she is still not happy that she had to make it:

> I placed Mom in January and I went through hell. The guilt was eating at me. I felt like I had committed the most violent of acts. How could I give up on Mom? I would have kept going and kept her at home, but that would have been more for me than her at this point.
>
> I woke up one morning to get her ready for day care and she started crying because she knew she was supposed to go somewhere but could not remember where or what she was supposed to do when she got there. Her fear level was so high I realized that moment that it was *time*. I could no longer keep her in my world as much as I wanted it.
>
> She has still not adjusted to being there. To this day, she tells everyone J. is coming to take me home. It is difficult, but in my heart and now in my head, I know I made the best decision for her and, as it turned out, for me as well.
>
> I still have bad days as I'm sure most people do, but not as severe as I used to. The loss is devastating, the guilt subsides a little, but the cloud over my head, for me anyway, will be there until Mom passes, whenever God decides it's time.
>
> Meanwhile, life goes on. I am a caregiver who gets no help from family, so it can be difficult. I am the only one, other than a couple of friends going in periodically, who visits Mom. I think I had to have at least twenty friends tell me I did the right thing before I finally was at peace with my decision.

M. has had extensive experience in nursing-home care, and her advice to gather information ahead of time is appropriate. We do make better decisions if we are informed and aware of our options:

> I would say ninety-nine percent of families feel guilty when they place their loved one in a nursing home. How the person will adjust is unpredictable. We have residents who were wild for the first night then just settled in nicely. We have others who were quiet and calm for the first few days then began to be restless. Many of our residents have daily needs to "go home," but even when our families take them "home" they still ask, "When can I go home?"
>
> Most of our admissions arrive after a recent crisis: illness or death of spouse, dangerous wandering, hospitalization, or aggression to family. I have noticed that the families are more accepting of placement if there has been a crisis. There seems to be a realization that they cannot do this on their own any more.
>
> As the saying goes, "There's no place like home," and a nursing home can never be a "home." There are good and bad nursing homes out there; there are no perfect ones. Do not rush your decision. Make sure that when the time comes you tour the place and see what goes on at the busiest time of the day. We do have to fill our beds to remain viable, and the good ones do have waiting lists.
>
> The right time is different for every family and every person with dementia. Many are cared for in the home until the end, but just don't let the disease consume you.

Peter's cynicism and concern about his mother are apparent in the following excerpt. Placing a loved one in the hands of competent caregivers doesn't seem to keep one from fretting. His mother's bridge is missing and he is critical of some aspects of her care, but he's realistic enough to know that some things will not be done to his satisfaction in a facility. Nonetheless, he is frustrated that he could not keep his mom at home. In his brusque, black-Irish way he tries to find humor—trying to hide the pain he feels:

> I went to see Mother today and noticed her bridge was still missing. I asked and they said, "Well, she had her tooth extracted and the bridge broke, and she may need more teeth removed." My mother is treated very well there, but this would never have hap-

pened a year ago. I would have been called. It was the way it was, but the unit is changing. Whether it's the new director, the cuts, the turnovers—I don't know.

My schedule is this: I see Mom once or twice a week and call the other nights. Eventually, whenever I called at night, no one would answer and by the time I could contact her she was in bed. I stopped calling.

Every time I come it's still rough. That's why I arranged the schedule I did. Timewise it was okay with her. We would sweet talk each other a little bit. The little, "I love you's."

"I love you, too."

"Are you okay?"

"Yes, Mom, I'm a little tired though." Then it was "guess time." Name the picture.

I made Mom a picture book of old and new pictures. They put these frames outside the door on small bulletin boards with an information card: name, city, family, and interests. The other night when I came to visit, we had our small talk and Mom says, "Blessed Mother, blessed Mother." So I think, "Okay, humm, church holiday?" No. She says again, "Blessed Mother, blessed Mother." So we go get an ice cream. What is life like without an ice cream cup? So we go back past her room. "Blessed Mother, blessed Mother." "Okay, Mom, yes, blessed Mother." So I look at the pictures and there is the one I took of her in front of the statue of The Blessed Mother. I laughed and shook my head. She had slipped one by me.

Today Agnes, her roommate, came by. She's eighty-eight and an ex-army nurse. I said hello as always, and she asked if I was her son or brother or maybe husband. Mom says "son." She tells me they used to be roommates. (They still are.) Agnes is neat because sometimes when I visit, she gives me a report like a nurse. "She's doing well and slept well," and she will always look you in the eye and touch Mom's shoulder while she's telling you. Its just like when you were a little kid and the doctor put his hand on your shoulder and said, "Well, I think he'll live." I think that's an official bedside manner rule.

Peter always closes his letters with a quote that somehow shows his anger and his pain. This time he closed with this: "W. C. Fields had a simple message for 'sunshine spreaders': 'Start every day off with a smile and get it over with.'"

When It's Right

The one thing about making decisions is that we can unmake some of them. Medicines can be altered and living accommodations changed. Some of the more difficult life and death decisions can't be altered, but let's talk about those more in the next chapter.

Carlene has wrestled with her decision to place her father and here is the result:

> . . . I have never been happy about the placement of my father in a facility. He has been living there, 165 miles from my home, for sixteen months now. Well, he is coming home in September and I am so excited I can hardly wait. I know it is the right thing to do as I am not feeling any dread or worry about it, just happiness.
>
> My father was placed because his care became more than my family and I could handle. He had been living with me for over five years. Dad was extremely active and never slept more than a few hours at a time. We had moved most of the furniture out of our house because he liked to tip things over. Well, he has changed considerably in the past months, and I don't think we will be dealing with those same problems. He is still able to walk but is not nearly as active as he was.
>
> Anyhow, I'm happy about this.

Obviously, this has been a painful decision for Carlene. We all hope that the next stage in her father's life will be easier on her and more satisfying for them all.

Dan Paris, formerly a social worker at Massachusetts General Memory Disorder Clinic and now a clinical social worker at Cabrini Medical Center in New York, gives us an insight from the perspective of both a family member and a professional dealing daily with placement decisions:

> One of the most frequent topics caregivers will ask questions about is long-term placement. Some families are curious as to whether the person they are caring for needs this permanent change. Other families have made a decision that a placement is needed, but are unsure as to when this should happen. When asked, I firmly endeavor to give a clear and concise response. Typically, I tell people "when it is right for your family."

Long-term placement is not a constant, but it is common. Most caregivers do not have the resources to be able to care for someone with Alzheimer's disease at home, particularly in the final stages. This is a difficult endeavor requiring almost constant supervision, significant environmental modifications, and frequent skilled care. It is unfortunate, but there is little insurance coverage available to family caregivers to fund these needs. So my experience is that most families will place their loved ones when that is the only way to get the level of care that is required.

Also, my experience is that placing a loved one is rarely easy. Some patients may be perfectly fine with the idea, but many are not happy about it. This is understandable. Their impairments from Alzheimer's disease are usually significant enough to mean they are really unable to understand why they must be placed. When, very early in the disease, many are able to recognize they are unsafe, I have seen several instances where people with Alzheimer's actually asked to move to assisted living. This is fortunate because many times patients are resistant. I have seen patients living alone forced out of their residences. This is never easy.

For my family, the decision was perhaps not too difficult. My grandmother's needs were quite clear, and she could not receive the level of care she required in my parents' house. She did attend a wonderful day program five days a week, and the family did the best it could with what it had, but it was not enough. I can honestly say that my professional opinion was also that Grandma needed a long-term placement. This did not make the decision easy.

One problem was the lack of adequate facilities. There were several wonderful assisted-living facilities I think Grandma would have done nicely in. Unfortunately, they were costly and were not covered by the Massachusetts Medicaid long-term-care benefit. Even though Grandma needed one of these Alzheimer's disease assisted-living residences, all Medicaid would pay for was a skilled nursing facility.

We looked at several places, and I think I armed my parents with a library of reading material. (I do have an office full after all.) The process took months between waiting lists and becoming comfortable with the decisions we made. The kicker was the trip to the emergency room. From there, it was actually smoother to have her move to the new facility. We did use a bit of a deception I suppose; several times the phrase "rehabilitation" was used. People with Alzheimer's sometimes become comfortable with being someplace new on their own accord for "rehabilitation." Many families will use these loving deceptions to help the process go more smoothly.

People always ask me which facility is a good one; I have actually had one or two caregivers wink at me while asking. I always hated the thought of a facility being chosen because "that damn social worker recommended it." So I usually give another "clear and concise response" to these questions and say "The one that works best for your family."

However, I almost always recommend that people put a patient into a facility with an Alzheimer's special care unit. Except for perhaps the very early stages where a normal assisted-living facility may be appropriate, these special care units should always be considered. They are not only wings in nursing homes, they are beautiful facilities in which I would have loved to have placed my grandma.

They have a physical layout designed for this disease with wander paths and color-coded walls. Their staffs are specifically and frequently trained in the very specialized skills of managing Alzheimer's disease. They have a lot of programming that takes into account the impairments of Alzheimer's disease, and patients are encouraged to participate. They usually genuinely understand what the patient's caregivers need. Many of these places go so far as to be very involved in any Alzheimer's event. They are great. They are also the ones that Medicaid will not cover.

The place we chose was a nursing home. Medicaid covers more nursing homes. It was clean, the staff was professional, and it did not smell. Smell is important. I advise all caregivers to put some stock in this sense when they judge a facility. One important difference was the Jewish cultural context that we thought Grandma would like. She had always been very involved in her Hadassah, and I felt it a safe bet that she would find the bingo she loved. My father felt it very important that he could also visit easily; this place was close.

This nursing home does have an Alzheimer's special care unit. Unfortunately, that is only for the most advanced patients; Grandma definitely did not belong there. So, she wound up on a wing that had several other Alzheimer's patients, but was not a special care unit. This has always made me nervous. Unfortunately, the staff on Grandma's wing has not received specific training in managing Alzheimer's disease that one would find in a special care unit. I don't blame the staff; I do blame their administration.

We made, I think, the best choices, taking into consideration not only the patient's needs, but the family's as well. I wish Grandma was in a special care unit, but I also wish Massachusetts Medicaid was a bit more sensible. Strangely, I have seen her more since she was diagnosed than the thirty-some-odd years prior to that time. It never ceases to amaze me how there can actually be positive experiences gained from facing Alzheimer's disease either as a patient or a caregiver.

Returning into the brambles of my mother's story, I know I made some poor choices:

- I waited too long to get her a thorough diagnosis.
- I tried to reason with her when there was no reason.
- I wasn't creative with her care.
- I didn't always consider all alternatives when making decisions.

Honestly, I didn't know all the alternatives. As a busy, working woman, I tended to take shortcuts; I regret I didn't have the patience I should have had.

I do believe the decisions I made for Mother's care were meant to be for her benefit. I know I tried not to do to her what I would not want done to myself. I am afraid, in all honesty, I sometimes acted for my benefit as well as hers, and if I could do it all over again, I would keep the Biblical injunction, "Do unto others . . ." close to my conscience.

Most of us remember Gilda Radner, whose comedic career ended with a painful cancer at too early an age. I have framed her words and have them above my computer as I write:

I wanted a perfect ending . . . Now, I've learned,
the hard way, that some poems don't rhyme,
and some stories don't have a clear beginning,
middle, and end. Life is about not knowing,
having to change, taking the moment,
and making the best of it, without knowing
what's going to happen next. Delicious Ambiguity.

Yes, I wanted it perfect.

NINE
With Every Goodbye We Learn

The Subject is Death

Caring for elderly family members goes back generations in Jean-Marie's family. Her grandfather had Alzheimer's in his early sixties and came to live with her family when she was quite young. He was there for sixteen years until he began falling and became more than her parents could manage. Jean-Marie remembers:

> My dad visited my grandfather every day, taking him to baseball games and out for sweets, reading to him, and sitting with him. He never missed a day and never went on vacation in case something happened to his father. At the end, my grandfather died of pneumonia, "the old people's friend."
>
> Now my dad is in the end stages of Alzheimer's. He has been hospitalized three times with pneumonia and speaks hardly at all. My dad began his Alzheimer's journey at age fifty-seven. He is now seventy-seven. It began when he couldn't remember if you stop for red lights or green lights. Then he couldn't remember where the school was—the school where he had taught for over twenty-five years. Dad was never aggressive, mean, or belligerent. He was mostly compliant, although at times he could be stubborn.
>
> This is the hardest and saddest stage of this terrible disease for me. I feel tremendous guilt for living far away and not being there

as often as I should. And then it happened. A few days prior to the time I had planned a trip home, Dad began putting out less urine and was moaning in pain. The nurse put him on liquid Tylenol and antibiotics. When I got home, I spent almost all my time just sitting next to my dad talking to him, holding his hand, rubbing him, playing his favorite music. He could barely speak and then only in whispers. I told him how much he meant to me and how much I loved him. I reminisced about all the things we did together.

His eyes were very bright, and he was eating quite well. He had this severe rattle in his chest and was having difficulty breathing. On Saturday we had a family supper with all the children, all of his brothers and sisters, and all of Mother's brothers and sisters. Before the evening ended each person went in and spoke with Dad, kissed him, or shook his hand. Shortly after that he got very agitated, breathing very heavily and looking panic-stricken. It took a long time to quiet him down. I kept holding his hand, saying it was okay, just relax and let go. He finally fell asleep.

Before I left for the airport the next morning, I sat with him again. His eyes were very alert and he ate all his breakfast. I gave him a kiss goodbye. He pulled on me to lean back down and he gave me a kiss and whispered with great difficulty, "I love you." It made my day. I blew a kiss from the doorway, and he blew one back. I left feeling it was a great visit. How lucky I was to have had time with him. The phone rang shortly after I got to my home to tell me that my dad had died in his sleep within an hour of my leaving.

I thank God for letting him live until we all got to say our goodbyes. I am sure Dad went in peace, knowing we all loved him so much.

When the subject is death, words die. Families bemoan the lack of available information to help them through these last times. Many caregivers are not even aware that hospice services are available to Alzheimer's patients. Honestly, many of us do not recognize the warning signs that tell us death is on its way, or perhaps we don't want to face the final finality. Just recently, the Alzheimer's Association published two brochures on the last stages, and information on hospice services is available through all of their chapters. Many Association chapters also conduct Last Stage support groups to help caregivers with the grief they feel and the knowledge they will need for this final stage. Still, much more is needed and most of us realize this—we know we need the knowledge to help us through this difficult time and yet we hide our heads and wish not to know. I guess that's just human. No one likes to hurt.

As our loved one's problems deepen, we depend upon physicians or hospital staffs to tell us what is available and warn us when our loved one reaches the final path of life. Perhaps because of our inclination to avoid discussing death, and perhaps because Death has his own schedule, these sources seem inadequate to the task. For one thing they know they may be wrong, and they don't want to alarm us needlessly. I can understand the hesitation. In my volunteer work I have not always been as forthright as I should have been, even though I heard the alarm bells ringing. We all—professional, semi-professional, and carers—stand waiting, with awe and trepidation, unsure and unwilling to say the dreaded name.

Reluctance to name the hour, however, doesn't keep us from being able to note symptoms that occur during the last stage of Alzheimer's. Although there is no typical scenario, there are signs that warn us that the disease is stealing still more abilities from our loved one's brain. Our loved one may begin to fall down for no apparent reason; he may have difficulty swallowing and, although we may puree food for him, he may clamp his jaws shut, refusing food or liquid. Sometimes a loved one will enter a coma and sometimes not. Aspiration pneumonia often will be the final end if he has ingested food that wrongfully enters the lung instead of the digestive tract.

Dena describes her experience:

> Mother had been battling pneumonia for about six months. She was having increasing difficulty swallowing, and she went to an all-liquid diet near the beginning of the summer. (In the last stage of Alzheimer's, many patients are unable to swallow, or try and choke on food causing pneumonia to develop.) In September, she had a bout that did not seem to respond to antibiotics. The cough did not clear up.
>
> We talked to the doctor who said that the pneumonias were *aspiration pneumonias* and were due to her swallowing difficulties. She advised us that they would keep recurring, and she asked us to think about whether to continue the treatments of antibiotics or whether we would let "nature take its course." Since we wanted hospice sup-

port, we eventually made the decision to NOT use antibiotics. They weren't helping anyway.

One Friday morning, Mom's caregiver, Shirley, got her up to give her a shower and things had changed. Mom was unresponsive. It was like she had turned a corner in whatever was left of her mind, and she decided she didn't want to live anymore. Shirley put Mom back to bed and called my sister and me about the change. Mom drank some of her milkshake that day, a little bit, but after that she refused any food. She clenched her teeth when anything was brought to her lips.

At that point we were okay with the decisions we had made, thinking that the end of Mom's long struggle was at hand. We had heard that "pneumonia is the old man's friend," ushering an old person out of the arena of suffering that they had been living in. Well, that week was hell. It wasn't easy for Mom, and it was hell to watch and hear. Mom's lungs filled with fluid, and there was nothing we could do. She was on morphine and Ativan. We kept her torso elevated. We had been told to swab her mouth out with a sponge, but even that seemed intrusive. She'd wrinkle her brow or chomp down on the swab. If it was too wet, it would drip down her throat and she would choke.

Most of the time Mom was unresponsive, but on Tuesday afternoon, after my middle sister flew in from Hawaii, Mom gathered her strength and opened her eyes for two periods, once for almost forty-five minutes. She struggled to communicate and made eye contact with us. We could not understand what she was trying to say, but it seemed important to her to make the effort. We'd read about this in the hospice materials and hoped that the end of mom's suffering would be soon.

Hospice expected her to die Tuesday. By that time her lungs were so full that when we lowered her bed to turn her or to change her clothes she would immediately start this terrible coughing. By Thursday everyone was exhausted. It had become a surreal existence of sleepless days and nights, deep introspection, and open talk between caregivers and family. I honestly thought that we were trapped in an endless doughnut of time, that my mother would just keep on going and outlast us all.

She died on Saturday morning, eight days after refusing all food and water. For us, pneumonia was not Mom's friend. I don't know what we could have done differently, but it sure seemed like she was suffering and there was not a damn thing I could do about it. By Thursday night, I wanted to pour the whole bottle of morphine down her throat, but she would have choked on it.

One of the hospice nurses said that Alzheimer's patients seem to take longer to die, because they are not able to "decide" to take that last breath. In the terminal stage of Alzheimer's, barring other medical problems, patients are so far gone that there is no free will remaining. So all of our talking to Mom and telling her it was okay to leave, that we would take care of each other, that she should leave her body behind and go join Dad and all her friends and be healthy again (go dance, Mom!), had no effect.

As the nurse said, with Alzheimer's patients, it comes down to a purely biological process. How long can the body hold out? Mom had been very well nourished. She wasn't emaciated, and so she lasted longer than I would have thought possible. I also secretly think that she had some really deep fear of the unknown, of opening that final door and knowing that there would be no way back.

I've been able to lock most of this away and examine it in very small pieces so that I don't break down. But it makes me so angry and upset and torn up that I couldn't have made it easier for her to die, after doing things to make it easier all through the long road of Alzheimer's. It haunts me when I think of it. I don't like feeling helpless. Perhaps it will just take more journal writing and long walks to absorb it all so that the memories aren't quite so raw.

The need for compassionate, knowledgeable medical advise is terribly important when we are dealing with death. However, truthfully, many physicians are reluctant to discuss the possibility of death and to tell the family what their options are. The words lay unspoken between us. At the end of treatment for my father's cancer, his oncologist simply told us he couldn't do anything more. We should call in hospice[1] services. We never heard from him again, not even a note. The same was true of the doctor who made the original diagnosis. As my mother lay in a coma in the nursing home, as far as I know, her doctor only talked to the nurses by phone; I never saw him and heard nothing until I called him after Mother's death and asked for a synopsis of what had happened. My contact with him was through the nurses at the home.

Here we are, engaged in one of the most important events of our lives, with medical personnel who apparently don't feel the need to educate us, a loved one we want to do our best for, not sure of what will happen next, and yet we may have to make some of the most profound decisions of our lives.

Our medical and legal experts have placed us in a position to have to almost single-handedly deal with the growing control we have over life. The control a Power of Attorney has over another human in the final symphony of life was made clear to me when I had to wield the baton for the ending coda to my mother's life. I had a Durable Power of Attorney, but Mother had no living will. I could only guess what her decisions would have been. She fell into a coma and she was not eating or taking in liquids. They asked if we wanted I.V.s started. Did we want to fight the infection that was taking her body? How far does a family go in prolonging human life? Do we want to resuscitate in case she stops breathing? Do we want a feeding tube? Do we want life support? These were the most difficult decisions I have ever had to make, and I felt completely alone. Unfortunately, today, most families have to find their own way around these decisions. To do that, we have to consider our personal view of life and death.

Why do we patiently bathe, rock, love, and massage these withered bodies with their withered brains? Why not do as we would an animal? A friend of my daughter's cynically said, when the nursing home staff asked her what to do about her Alzheimer's mother, "If she were my dog, I'd consider euthanasia." All things considered, why do so many, many caregivers desperately look for anything that will extend that fractured life? We take them for walks, put them on fat-free diets. Why bother? Alzheimer's is a death sentence, so why allow them to continue to suffer? Put them out of their misery. How many times have we heard fellow caregivers bemoan the condition of their loved one. "He is not really alive, he might as well be dead." "She has no quality of life."

Carol B. has given this a lot of thought:

> Alzheimer's is a long, slow death. The body remains intact long after the mind; spirit and essence seem to have departed, at least by all outside appearances.
>
> So when the body begins to fail, in some way or another, death, from whatever cause, is in fact the natural process of ending the journey and letting the body depart also. It seems to me that using

medical intervention at that point is exerting man's will, not God's will. Intervention would be a man-made interference with the natural process of dying. It is not something I want done on my mother's behalf; her death has been far too long in coming and will be a final release she has so long deserved.

Asking for a no-code or "do not resuscitate" order is not, in my belief, ending another's life; it is letting God, or nature, or whatever one believes, take the final step of letting the people we love leave their sickly bodies and go home.

While at first I had some reservations about the *rightness* of withholding a feeding tube, I have no such doubts now. When my mother's body refuses to take sustenance on its own, it will be the beginning of the long-awaited release I have hoped for so long. Inserting a feeding tube would seem more like a subversion of God's will than an act of kindness.

Today we *can* prolong life, almost indefinitely, and we also have the legal power to withhold substances that will help to lengthen life. When is *the* moment when life no longer has meaning and should be ended? Is it when they don't know us or know their own names? Is it when they are incontinent? Is it when they actually *ask* for the "black pill," indicating their desire to die? Is it when they endure too much suffering, or is it when it is right and convenient for us? When does life lose its meaning and become only a suffering agony? When is the right time to end it? I can't answer these questions for myself, let alone others, but the mere fact that they are present indicates a need to proceed with caution when we are so deeply involved in another's life. It is an awesome responsibility.

Nothing I had read prepared me for that week when my own mother died. I don't know if anything can prepare one for the death of a loved one. Caregivers call for more and more information on the last stage of this disease, and yet we are never prepared and seldom want to hear those words of finality. It isn't just the final hours, it's the weeks and months leading up to them that are so difficult. The built-up stress leaves you unprepared for these difficult last days. When the end finally comes you feel that it simply can't be happening. Families walk around as in a time warp, often unable to complete the easiest tasks or answer the simplest questions.

At my father's death I was so focused on his pulse (I had my left hand in his armpit and my right hand holding his other hand) that nothing could have gotten my attention. And nothing could have pulled me from my post. My world had become his and I was wrapped in some sort of deathwatch. As he breathed, I breathed. I don't remember what anyone else was doing; it was just the two of us locked in some timeless ritual.

When Mother was in the final stage of Alzheimer's, I desperately wanted someone to put her out of her misery. It is so heartbreaking to watch the slow dissolution of a proud human life. I could not understand a God who would allow anyone to suffer as she did. The first symptom was a urinary tract infection that seemed impossible to clear up. The nursing home staff warned me that she was quite ill and probably didn't have more than two weeks to live. Given antibiotics, she recovered and lived a few more weeks. Then she began to fall; she fell frontward, sideways, backwards; she fell in hallways, out of wheelchairs, out of Geri chairs, into people and out of bed. Her eighty-six-year-old body was a solid bruise. When she spoke to me I saw that even her tongue was bruised. Who would want to prolong such agony?

However, for my mother, this prelude of pain was followed by a kind of peace. There is a quality of human life that the Greeks called *arête,'* human virtue or excellence. In our Western culture this virtue is often present at the time of death. In Shakespeare, how a man dies tells something about the man; it finalizes the character of the person. Horatio, in *Hamlet,* cries out, *"Good night, sweet prince: and flights of angels sing thee to thy rest."* All of this is to say that death is an important part of a person's life and our departure is as important to life's symphony as our entrance.

When I think of Mother's death, I think of the quote, "When it's dark enough, men see the stars." Shortly before her final sleep began, Mother looked up at me, kissed me, and she knew who I was for the first time in two years. In a clear voice and with a clear mind, my mother asked me, "Am I dying?" And then she told me she loved me and gave me the warmest hug any daughter could have. Within a few hours she fell asleep and never awoke, but in that moment of clarity I witnessed the *arête* in my mother's being. My mother was there! She, not the Alzheimer's person I had been seeing, but my *real* mother, had survived that horribly painful, fracturing disease. At the moment of death, *she*, not the changed human being who had taken her place, was present. What courage and strength it had taken for her to fight that battle. To this day I'm not sure why this trial was asked of her, but when she left us, what was lost was the pure gold of my mother's being.

After five days in a coma, my mother died in the middle of the night, and I was not with her.

The Grief Goes On

The finality of death takes our breath away. We weren't nearly as ready as we thought we would be. Suddenly I had all these questions to ask Mother, none of which would ever be answered. I was angry at my decision to leave her that night and angry with the nurses for telling me her vital signs were good. If I had been warned, I would have been with her, but I wasn't, and it still breaks my heart. Another bad decision. No, we are never ready to let go; there is always one last thought to share, one final act of love to show, and when we can no longer do this, we weep and pine for lost opportunities.

But there are comforting thoughts that, unbidden, come to soothe the wounds of loss. Michele writes of her mother's final days:

> Mother said repeatedly that she wanted to go home. And in the last couple of days she cried quietly while saying this. She wanted her mother. Later, she said she had seen her mother. When I asked what her mother had said, she told me, "Nothing." This actual sighting of her mother seemed so different from her former thoughts. Later she asked where her husband was. (Michele's father had died six months before this.) Again, I assured her that he would return later. Aside from her bath and the headache/neckache that had plagued her for a few days, she had such a good day, I thought, calmer, resting peacefully. She told me at least a dozen times how beautiful I was, this woman who really couldn't see any longer, but to me the words were priceless. As I left she gave me her "blessing" instead of the usual plea for my return.

I've felt so privileged to have taken care of my parents. When I started, it was a "job." But somewhere into the journey, I found love with these people who called me their first child. They would have celebrated their fiftieth anniversary a couple of weeks ago; now they are celebrating together.

Of all the caregivers I have known, none has walked away unscathed by the death of their loved one, regardless of the amount of grieving done along the way. Euphoria may carry us over the initial shock, and it may take a while for us to realize that we can't collect our thoughts, we feel at loose ends and we're not sure just yet where the future lies.

- We find our thoughts going ever backward as we try to bring some closure to the event. Tasks are undone and tears come quickly when we review our own actions. Did we help our loved one die with dignity? Did we handle the rituals of death correctly? Did I give the kind of caregiving I would want for myself? We feel a deep need for someone to tell us we "did it right."
- We may dream about our loved one's death or about her returning to us with messages.
- We find ourselves unable to get off the Alzheimer's cul-de-sac, because we are still focused in a carer's mindset. We go past friends and family with that vacant look that takes in the world and yet sees nothing. We are absent souls and our eyes reveal this. They say, "Nobody home."
- Memories of the one who is gone return unbidden—some of them sweet and tender, others requiring further thought before we can deal with them. We may begin to analyze the complexities of our relationship with the one who is gone.
- Finally, we realize we haven't healed—we're only mending.

Deep in December it's nice to remember,
Without a hurt the heart is hollow.
—Tom Jones, *Try to Remember*

My father died of cancer in 1986, and Mother died in 1996 after eight years of Alzheimer's. Both deaths are as fresh in my mind today as they were then. I know they are a part of my being, and I will never forget. I can never return to being the person I was prior to witnessing their deaths, but the blackbirds do continue to sing, and life does go on.

A grandchild's birth, a walk in the fall leaves. Memories of earlier, happier days with my parents are also part of the web of life. A certain pink rose grows in my garden, and every year when it blooms (always the last rose of summer) it is a precious memory of my father. He loved that particular rose. A grandson is born, and my son names him after his grandfather. And the ice in my heart melts a little more.

I visit my memories of them, now and then, and deal with the feelings that come. I return to pay a visit and grapple with the events that have hurt my family and me so deeply. It is part of the mending process. I have learned not to be afraid to hurt. Hurting is part of life. I have learned to get all the help I need in order to mend, and I have learned to ask others to help me at times of crisis. I no longer feel a need to be perfect.

As a result I'm beginning to remember the happier side of Mother and her illness and the times we cuddled and shared "I love you" with one another. I have learned to listen to others to be curious about Alzheimer's and less of afraid of it, and I learned that whatever I did wrong was because I cared too much and I was afraid—afraid almost to the point of being frozen in time.

I was so serious, so tense, so hurting and unrelentingly bound to the struggle. I guess I thought my struggle would help Mother survive longer, but it didn't. Perhaps I felt that if I just gave enough of myself to the fight, I could lick this thing. When Mother had a good day, I would think we could win, only to be sent once more into the pit when she had a bad day. I could never cure her, never make her happy, and I seldom did the right thing at the right time. Now I know that no one can do these things.

What I did give Mother was the gift of love. After all my attempts to get through to her damaged brain, I finally gave up, and all I could do was love her, hold her, and hope she felt my warmth. I failed her in so many ways, but I loved her and learned to show it as I relaxed with the disease.

The Pillars of Care

Sometimes, as the saying goes, we have to "Let go and let God." Education, research, support, and attention to one's own health are four of the most important pillars of Alzheimer's care. They will help us survive this evil disease, but a fifth is "rolling with it," and a sixth is "a sense of humor." None of us will live according to these supports 100 percent of the time, but I wish I had worried less and laughed and hugged Mother more. Ah, me! Hindsight.

I want the last words in this chapter to be devoted to one of my favorite Alzheimer's professionals, Geri Hall. Her words are wise and true:

> Alzheimer's changes you forever. Some ways it changes you are bad. It robs you of health and sleep. It teaches you about grief more intimately than you ever expected; it teaches you that for all your qualities, you have fatigue, temper, and anger at the one you love more than anyone else.
>
> But, too, it brings out a depth of feeling most people never feel, it teaches you joy at small things, the ability to touch others with your soul, and to value each good moment you have. It teaches you to practice politics, to feel compassion for weakness, and to understand that we are not given the gift of control, so we can let go from time to time.

With every goodbye we heal.

PART TWO

WHAT'S IT LIKE TO BE . . . ?

Introduction to Part Two:
What's it Like to Be...?

The Family

This is the nest in which soul is born,
nurtured and released into life. It has
an elaborate history and ancestry and a
network of unpredictable personalities
—grandparents, uncles, aunts, cousins.
Its stories tell of happy times and tragedies.

—Thomas Moore

The nests provided by families are as dissimilar as the members within those families. How will an individual react to a mother's disease? No one knows until it happens. How will children or grandchildren weather a crisis? No one knows before the fact. These are the complexities that make life so interesting and yet so unpredictable and sometimes appalling. Some family members are drawn closer to the family structure by tragic events, and others want nothing more than to leave the scene and avoid the pain and anguish. Siblings can join together for family strength or wage war with one another to gain control of an uneasy situation.

How family members react often depends upon the myths and history of the family, the teachings of guilt, duty, responsibility, love, and family unity all enter into and influence what happens. And then, too, personal emotional responses of family members can affect the picture, and traditions are thrown out the window, resulting in a knee-jerk reaction at the time of the tragedy. We see events through our own private prisms and emotionally a family can ricochet off of one another, causing a lack of focus and stability at a time when slow and steady is the best plan of action. We are all loose cannons in a time of crisis and no one can predict what will happen, nor can we predict how the event will change family members or the family as a whole.

Rachel Remen is a doctor and counselor to cancer patients. She has observed "that people with the same disease have very different stories . . . Their stories were as different as their fingerprints." When someone tells their story it is from their personal viewpoint and not, as Dr. Remen says, "the experience itself . . . Truth is highly subjective. This is what makes family stories precious: they escape the objective view of the moment and concentrate, instead, on what a human being involved in the drama is feeling and thinking. This is where we glimpse the human condition." Generalities are out (*Kitchen Table Wisdom* xxvii).

Thanks to the kindness of those who have shared their experiences, the stories in the next three chapters offer a wider, more intense view of seven different families affected by Alzheimer's. In the previous chapters we concentrated more on specific times in a caregiver's experience. The following stories are designed to provide us with a view, over time, of the effects of Alzheimer's on a family through the eyes of one family member. What were their problems? How did they handle the Alzheimer's intruder? What was there in the family history that influenced how they dealt with the disease? What did they learn as a result of their ordeal?

Seldom are we permitted such an intense look at what usually happens in private, and I want to personally thank those who have shared their stories with us. We learn best by imitation and experience; through these experiences, our own private worlds may be strengthened and enriched.

TEN
Children in the Family

Nothing that grieves us can be called little:
by the eternal laws of proportion a
child's loss of a doll and a king's loss
of a crown are events of the same size.
—Mark Twain

Sara's Story

What is it like to be a thirteen-year-old granddaughter in a home where Grandma is well into her Alzheimer's years? Sara lived with her brother, sister, grandmother, and parents in Connecticut at the time she wrote this paper for a class project:

> Alzheimer's is a terrible disease. My Grandma Rose has had it for a long time; in fact I can barely remember my grandma for who she really was. She is covered by a shell that never lets the feelings and emotions she once had show. She is not the grandma that I remember.
>
> My grandma was such a wonderful person, so filled with life. I remember when I was very young, my grandma would make me waffles. She did many things for me because she loved me. Today she no longer recognizes me even when I tell her my name.
>
> My grandma Rose has changed so much, as people often do. Her hair is short and silver. Her eyes are quiet and empty. Her face, once flushed with life, is now expressionless. Her anger and frustration no longer seem to be a part of her. She sits aimlessly staring into a world we can no longer reach. How I miss the warm smiles of love and recognition toward my family and myself. Many of her habits are becoming quite annoying. She sings songs all day, most are just combinations of words. She can never seem to keep her body or hands still.

I am the oldest girl in my family, so I have the responsibility of helping my mother care for my grandma. Occasionally, I have to change her diapers, feed her, and bathe her. When she first came to our house about two years ago, I thought she was disgusting. I have matured since then, and now I realize that it is not fair to say that about her. She is not disgusting because what she has become is not her true self.

My little sister Rachel is seven. She has always been very special to me. I have been concerned with her lately because she seems far away. Her work in school has been suffering because of her troubled mind. She understands that our grandmother is not going to get better, and I believe that this constant stress is her problem.

My brother Matthew is fifteen and never helps care for our grandma. He refuses to see her nude. I respect that, but sometimes I get so angry because he will never help me with her.

Lately, my mother has been having more trouble with her. This lady is her mother . . . or should I say this "being" is her mother? I love my mother very much, and I can feel the pain that she feels every day. My mother also knows that she might possibly be next in line for this disease. It is a disease that no one wants to get. She does not want her family to suffer. She knows that our family is having enormous trouble with Grandma and does not want our future families to go through what we are now.

My father deals with my grandma the best he can. He helps change her diapers and feeds her, just as he did for me when I was a baby. My father said, "It is a shame that someone you love and who is so vibrant and personable becomes a non-person."

I know that I have to face reality. My sister, my mother, my brother, and I all run the risk of getting this disease. It is a very scary thought. We must live our lives and not worry. Hopefully, God will spare us from this dreadful disease.

As the years pass, my grandma slowly wastes away. I hope that God will soon take her. She is not getting better, but much worse. It makes me sad to see the grandma that shared so much love with me slowly dying. I only pray to God that she is truly happy in her own world.

We comfort ourselves with the belief that children adapt and adjust, but I'm not sure this is true when the pain is Alzheimer's. Reading between the lines we can feel Sara's fear that this terrible thing might happen to her and to other members of her family. She is concerned for her parents and siblings and the effect Alzheimer's is having on them as a family unit.

Wisely, she knows that her grandmother cannot control what is happening to her, but she is very aware of the emotional stress that Grandma's care is causing her family. Interestingly, not once does Sara voice the opinion that they should find a home for Grandma. Obviously, home care for Grandma is an accepted, important project for this family while other families might place Grandma in a care facility rather than endure the stress and depression it puts on the family. What is *right?* These are decisions only a family can make.

Sara's story reveals something about Sara: part of her grief is the loss of love she feels as her grandmother has abandoned her role in Sara's life. Like many caregivers, Sara associates Grandma not recognizing her with a loss of love, and it hurts. She cherishes the memories of her *hands-on* grandmother of the past, but is still unable, or perhaps unwilling, to love the Alzheimer's grandmother. Perhaps time will allow her to celebrate this part of Grandma's Alzheimer's life as well as the years that preceded it.

Families caring for loved ones in a home in which children or teens are present usually are aware of the responsibility this entails; the need to discuss life, death, pain, sorrow, and love with the younger members of the family can not only help them through the event, but provide a foundation, an undergirding of strength for the future.

J.'s Story

Today, J. is an artist who lives with her family in a peaceful country environment. Now life is good; her family, her studio, and her horses make up a pleasant life, but she realizes that her childhood experiences have caused her problems in her adult life. She explains *what is it like* to be the child of an early-onset Alzheimer's patient:

> My dad died of probable Alzheimer's several years ago after being symptomatic since my earliest memories. Now my concern is that since this was what they call early-onset, that there is a great chance it is familial. Unfortunately, there was no autopsy, and I know nothing about his family.

The fear and assumption that I would get the disease has influenced how I have lived my life. Now I have reached the age I never expected to see, and I'm really amazed I'm still of sound mind. I wonder if my partner might soon find himself looking after me alone. At any rate, my fears are not why I write. I'm writing to show the other side of life in an Alzheimer's family: children caught in a strange dream.

When Dad started to exhibit symptoms of dementia there was not yet much talk of Alzheimer's. He was forty-three when I was born, and I can't remember a time when he didn't have periods of helplessness and confusion. He would go into these mysterious rages about what seemed to be nothing, but we were very isolated and I didn't know that wasn't normal. We didn't think there was anything wrong with him, we just thought he was an asshole. At least none of the doctors we knew mentioned what was causing his behavior. His illness was a guilty family secret. Imagine my guilt, fear, and embarrassment when, at the age of twelve, my teachers would call home to complain about my truancy or my behavior and find that my father didn't know who I was. Or imagine him just talking nonsense or simply breathing into the phone. I had a time making up lies to cover that.

I remember that Mother only realized, or admitted, that there was something really wrong when he started to have very bad vision problems and refused to admit it. He would get up around five in the morning and steal Mother's glasses so he could read whatever he needed to read when no one would see him. Then he'd forget and leave her glasses in the fridge. When confronted, he denied it all.

I left home at fifteen in order to escape it all, and when I returned home at seventeen, I remember Mother wanted my help in placing him in a nursing home. He had attacked the landscape workers who came to cut our lawn and weed our gardens with an axe. They had made it to their truck and shut the door before he caught them, but he had taken the axe to the truck before they had made it out of the driveway.

My mother treated my father with obvious contempt and impatience. I suppose there must have been compassion there because physically she looked after him very well, but to a child it sure wasn't a visible kindness. What I thought I saw was hatred. Her anger usually took the form of verbal, psychological, and physical abuse of me. She was extremely violent toward me. My father was violent

too, but not towards me, and you could see in his eyes that his out-
bursts were brought on by confusion and terror.

I'll spare you any more graphic descriptions. I read an article last
week in which a lady stated that she didn't resent her mother's dependence any more than her mother had resented her as a baby. I always assumed that people hated adults who became dependent. Had
I realized that there could be understanding about demented people, I wouldn't have lived the first half of my life feeling that Alzheimer's would be the worst possible fate. It's not the disease I feared
but the contempt, fear, and hatred that I thought always went with
it. This is a good reason for public education and awareness.

J.'s comment about her family not knowing her father was ill has been
true of many early-onset victims. Until recently, Alzheimer's was seldom
contemplated as a cause of dementia in younger patients. Every other
illness and emotional quirk was considered first. What we have often labeled "meanness" may have been due to underlying mental and chem-
ical conditions.

And did you hear that bell ring in her last paragraph? Part of the fear
of Alzheimer's is the fear of ridicule, contempt, and hate. This is how she
saw her father treated, and she assumed this was the attitude all persons
have toward the mentally disabled. Add to this a mother so beset with
financial and emotional worries that she lets out her angry feelings on
her children. Here are human beings stretched to the limits of their love
and capabilities. I can't help but ask: what kind of education and help can
a society offer to those who are stretched beyond their abilities to cope?

Saddest of all is the fact that the most driven of all these families are
the ones we have the most difficulty reaching. They are persons who do
not look to others for help—persons who do not believe that society has
any answers for them. They are not apt to call the Alzheimer's Association for help. They make do. They exist. They cope, not always well,
but they cope. The only times we reach them is if one ends up in a
homeless shelter or if authorities are called in at a time of crisis. They
don't understand how to manipulate the system, and their family myth
tells them to take care of their own. They are outside the avenues of social programming. They are unseen—sometimes bitter, sometimes
combative, sometimes unreasonably and unhealthily placid. Always this
is sad, for even though social agencies may be able to treat for the mo-

ment, the long-term programs needed to solve such ingrained family problems are just not present.

Leslie's Story

What is it like to be falling in love and, at the same time, watching your grandmother slowly fade away? It's like looking at the alpha and omega of the human condition before we are old enough to make these comparisons.

The year I met my husband my grandmother forgot who she was. I met Mitch in May, a month before my parents would lead my dimming grandmother out of the house forever. She would leave the home where for twenty years, she had lived with my mother and father and helped raise her grandchildren to leave and make lives of their own. That bright June day she stood on the front porch, looked back over her shoulder. She took in every detail, sighed deeply, and went with my parents, trusting.

Married when she was seventeen, two months shy of her eighteenth birthday, Mammaw had loved Pappaw fiercely in the way of a child bride, a devoted woman-girl who looked to him to smooth all paths, to solve the impenetrable mysteries of money, insurance, and taxes. In return, she teased him out of foul moods, laid out his clothes, and bathed him when he could no longer do it for himself. One night when I was a teenager, I wandered downstairs to watch TV and found my grandmother sitting on his lap giggling like a young girl.

"Did you ever kiss Pappaw before you married?" I asked my grandmother at lunch one day.

"No, I never did."

She was expert and practiced at such little white lies, and we often wondered if her fears and fibs didn't fold into themselves, leaving her mind a tangled, whimsical origami.

Following my grandfather's death, her illness came on like a long rolling storm, gathering dark woolen clouds, until the light in her eyes began to recede. Months after his passing, my mother found Mammaw sitting downstairs in the dark, staring into the darkening room. "Do you ever cry for him?" my mother asked. Mammaw, her eyes wide, hands twisting a tissue into shreds, shook her head. "I try to be a good girl."

Three years later on Christmas Eve of my grandmother's seventy-ninth year, she called me downstairs to help her decide how much money to give my parents as a gift. She asked if $200 would be enough, and I said I thought it was very generous.

"How do you write that?"

"What?"

"How do you write $200?"

Puzzled, I guided her while she wrote the check.

Deep down, we knew what was happening. We knew in our hearts Mammaw was beginning a journey—a journey that minute by minute would take her to a place where we couldn't go. It was months before any of us could say the word Alzheimer's.

That June my parents placed my grandmother in a nursing home called Bear Creek, fifteen minutes from their house, where, if you stood on your toes on the front lawn, you could see the burnt orange rock formations made famous in Colorado postcards. At the time it was one of the few facilities in the area that took Alzheimer's patients; like wind-up toys released in different directions, they were too hard for many nursing homes to contain.

The staff in the Alzheimer's ward was as warm and sweet as bread pudding, cuddling these loopy seniors like frightened five-year-olds on their first day of school. They posted tiny biographies outside patients' doors—life maps to the twilight zone, which read eerily like living obituaries. Sylvie was a homemaker who lived in suburban Denver. She raised three children, had five grandchildren, and she enjoyed gardening, cooking, and spending time with family. Ed was a postal carrier who was married with two children. He retired in 1973, the same year his wife died of cancer. He enjoyed building model trains and woodworking. Elma was a homemaker and antique dealer. She is now a widow and has one daughter and two grandchildren. She enjoyed going to church and traveling back home to Indiana.

But the social workers and the vinyl sofas done up in mauves and teals did little to conceal the fact that this was not a home but a place of waiting. These sweet befuddled souls who didn't know their names or the names of their children, knew they had been exiled, snatched from their quilts and delft and honey-I-love-you's.

Wandering up and down the linoleum in their orthopedic shoes, Mammaw's neighbors screamed to go home or punched friends in fits of pique. One woman in her sixties walked the halls clicking her teeth like castanets. Gladys, in cat-eye glasses and clutching her purse, demanded, "Where's my son? Take me home!" Another woman yelled "help" every three seconds, as if this personal tic would engender the aid she really needed.

When I visited Bear Creek, Mammaw clutched my arm at any sign of leaving, begging me to take her home to the braided rug in her bedroom, to the bottle of Chanel No. 5 on her dresser, to the navy blue dress—her elopement dress—she kept in a box. "You *are* home, Mammaw," I'd say, understanding that even the shadows couldn't conceal my lie or our mutual heartbreak.

By the time Mitch, my "to be" husband, came along, I knew a man must know the facts and details of a woman's life. The night we met, the rain reflecting the lights of the city into jewels, I told him that I had been raised by my parents *and* by my grandparents and how I loved the upbringing which had skewed my values from that of my peers. He looked at me, head tilted shyly, a slight smile chasing his face, and talked of his love for his Papa Louis and of his family flung from one end of the country to the other. When he asked for my phone number, I handed him my card, which he earnestly tucked into his wallet. I never, ever doubted he would call.

Shortly after my grandmother's diagnosis, Mitch and I went to a budget showing of "Driving Miss Daisy." Pictured in the nursing home at the end of the film, the neatly regimented Miss Daisy sat hunched over her lunch, her hair a blowzy, confused aura; she looked smudged as if part of her had been erased. My grandma, who had always worn her hair in a chic French roll, padded the floor of her new home, her hair a cacophony of short, truncated curls like she had been scribbled out.

Not long after that night, I took Mitch to meet my grandmother. She was sitting on her bed, pulling the drawer of her nightstand in and out. The wreath I had made for her one Mother's Day hung on the wall, its periwinkle bow slightly askew. "Mammaw," I said, sitting next to her. "This is my boyfriend, Mitch."

"Clint?" she asked, her eyes cloudy and dim.

"No, not Pappaw. This is Mitch."

"Mish?"

"That's right."

Looking at his handsome face, she grabbed his arm like a life preserver in a stormy sea.

"On a hill far away, stood an old rugged cross," she hummed. "A symbol of suffering and shame. . . . You remember that one don't you?" And Mitch, a Jewish man holding her arm like a prince at the ball, paraded her down the long linoleum passage. "You bet, Grandma. You bet."

Three years later when I walked down the aisle, escorted by my parents, I walked with many ghosts: friends long dead, my grandfather gone seven years, and Mammaw, whose personality lay in our hearts and memories while her shell still wandered the day room. The sun shown resolute and bright that afternoon, its benediction of warmth and flowers linking this day to all other sun-blessed days.

At the end of the ceremony, Mitch crushed the glass under his foot, and we turned to face the people we loved. A handful of chairs sat empty in the dappled, yellow light.

Children raised under the cloud of Alzheimer's must accept those empty chairs long before death takes their loved ones away. As an Alzheimer's family, it is the curse we live with. Leslie is my daughter, and reading this over brings great tears of remembrance to my eyes, a sadness that she had to experience such grief at such a happy time in her life.

Leslie was a stalwart, gallant, and loving granddaughter, and I don't think I was ever more proud of her than during her grandmother's Alzheimer's years. Our family, my mother and father, my husband and myself, and our two children lived together for many years. The closeness of my children and my parents has proved to be a mixed blessing: on one hand, it has given my children a serious, thoughtful approach to life and a deep closeness to their grandparents, on the other hand, they have realized early the full pain of close loss, of empty chairs.

ELEVEN
The Smudged Years

> *It often seems as though the families of
> Alzheimer's patients are sidetracked from
> the broad sunlit avenues of ongoing life,
> remaining trapped for years, each in its
> own excruciating cul-de-sac. The only rescue
> comes with the death of a person they love.
> And even then, the memories and the
> dreadful toll drag on, and from these
> the release can only be partial.
> A life that has been well lived and a shared
> sense of happiness and accomplishment are
> ever after seen through the smudged glass of
> its last few years. For the survivors the
> concourse of existence has forever
> become less bright and less direct.*
>
> —Sherwin B. Nuland, *How We Die*

What can we expect from "the smudged glass" years? There are huge differences in what each family experiences, "each in its own excruciating cul-de-sac." But most will tell you they feel a sense of being apart from normal life and social concerns during these caregiving times and admit that the smudged glass of the last years dominates their memories of their loved one.

These years take on a personality of their own, leaving the family having difficulty reconstructing the real person they have lost. Sometimes they find they are even unable to reconstruct themselves. This chapter looks at two families. The first story introduces us to Billie Beatrice, whose bout with Alzheimer's lasted for twenty years; the second account tells of a reconciliation between a father and daughter during the smudged years.

Billie Beatrice

What is it like to be the daughter of a mother who has had Alzheimer's for two decades? What kind of mindset do you have to have to endure this?

Early-onset Alzheimer's disease accounts for up to ten percent of the total Alzheimer's patient toll. With an estimated four million patients in the United States diagnosed with the disease, this means that approximately 400,000 of them are coping with the problems of early-onset Alzheimer's. It usually starts before age sixty-five and sometimes as early as forty or fifty. Sometimes it runs a rapid course, taking the person in a few years, but if the patient's overall health is good, he or she may live for a very long time (Living with Early-onset Alzheimer's Disease 1–2).

Carol writes a sad note about a visit to her mother's nursing home:

> I just returned from seeing my mother in the nursing home 350 miles from me. My mother is in her nineteenth year of Alzheimer's; she developed early-onset at age fifty-two and just turned seventy-two as this was written. My mother is Billie Beatrice, and I am her daughter Carol.
>
> This has been going on for so long that I am no longer shocked or surprised, or even angered, by anything I see. But it is so depressing. I didn't even cry this time; maybe I've become somewhat inured to the pain of seeing her in this condition. She's been in the nursing home for eight years.
>
> My mother can't speak at all. The last time I heard her say even yes or no was five years ago. That's five years of silence! Seven years ago she could still say "I love you," which she said to anyone near her, but for the last four years she only makes sounds like grunts and groans. As I watch her lying there, I wonder if her agony is screaming the same thought to her.
>
> Almost nothing is left of my wonderful mother with the vibrant red hair. The hair, still thick and full but white, is almost all there is left. She is curled into a fetal position, both of her hands clutched in little balls to her upper chest, absolutely immobile and rigid. One of her legs is curled upright in about a forty-five-degree angle, also immobile and rigid.
>
> The nursing staff has posted two diagrams next to her bed on how and where to position pillow bolsters around her feet, legs, and

between her knees. They are trying to slow the continuing compression of her body into a rigid fetal position because they fear that trying to move her limbs to bathe, move, and clothe her will cause her physical pain while doing so.

She makes regular grimaces and contortions of her face, grinding her teeth in a highly audible way. Her eyes wander constantly and don't seem to fix upon anything. I don't believe she sees me—by that I mean I can't see any recognition at all, even to know if she's aware of the body of the human before her. She doesn't seem to respond to any sounds, but I'm not completely sure of that. All of this has been pretty consistent for the last three years.

And the really bad news is that she has not developed any additional specific physical problems like bronchitis or pneumonia or something that might hasten her leaving this tortured state and going to the God she has always loved. In fact, while reviewing her chart with the nurses, I found out she has gained six pounds, up from 102 to 108. The nurses say she still has a good appetite.

On this visit, she starts doing something new. She tries to raise her head above her pillow. Consider the effort and literal pain in the neck it must cause to continually try to raise your head an inch or so above your pillow, and again I want to ask God why can't he take her now. At my request, one of the nurses elevated her bed, but she still kept trying to raise her head.

I lotioned her body, checked her legs and hips, still no sores of any kind. I am so grateful to the nursing staff for that. This disease is also difficult for professional caregivers. They still remember her singing goodnight to all the residents on the unit when she first came to the nursing home so long ago. They hurt with us.

I combed her hair; massaged her head, neck, and shoulders; cleaned her ears; cleaned her nose; clipped and filed her nails; and got my fingers intertwined into hers, watching to see if there would ever be any cognition in her eyes. It was not that she knew ME— that went away many, many years ago—but just maybe she would know it was someone important to her who was there with her. It didn't happen. That hurts so much.

At the end of my visit, I asked my younger brother, who was there with me, if he would leave the room for a few minutes. To be honest, I had such an impulse to take her pillow and put an end to this hell on earth that she's in. I can't of course. More for my benefit than for hers, I could not live with such an act.

What I did do was hold her head and put my face directly in front of hers, so she could see nothing else, and talked to her about leaving, letting go, going to God, and being my guardian angel from the better place I believe she deserves. I talked to her about leaving now and leading the way for all of us to find her later.

And then I noticed that her eyes were wet with tears! I brushed them off, but they came back, again and yet again until I had to believe what I was seeing: she was crying, they were real tears. Now I am carrying a heavy stone in my heart at the thought that she still feels emotional pain.

Would you all add a brief request to your prayers and ask that God bring Billie Beatrice home?

Carol was about forty at the time this was written, so almost half of her life had been deeply affected by having a demented mother. She mentioned several times the fear she had that her mother was locked in a body that refused to react—what if Billie knew what was happening to her but could not communicate? Add to that the difficulty of trying to keep her mother alive in her memory and for twenty years having to watch the deterioration of that memory, and it is not difficult to realize the impact this has had on Carol.

"God, now I feel like crying. You know what I mean?" Carol says. Continuing, she gives us some added information about her mother's life:

I cannot forget the first time I visited Mother in the nursing home and heard her caterwauling and saw her strapped in a vest that was strapped to a Geri chair that was strapped to a table. In her all-too-visible agitation, she was moving both the chair and the table forward. When I rushed to grasp her hand, she yanked me to her so tightly I almost fell. Her strength and determination floored me. As I talked to her, stroking her hand while I asked the R.N. about her medications, she became utterly calm, even serene, and did not make a sound. I don't believe she doesn't feel things inside.

And it isn't just my mother. It has completely changed my father's life, too, very directly. It has affected all of us: her children, her grandchildren, her siblings, and her good friends. Almost everything the two of them worked for together is gone. They became innocent bystanders of the crime against humanity known as Alzheimer's.

They married young, worked hard to support the five children they had, and lived as good, taxpaying citizens struggling to buy their first home. They were middle-class Americans, working to get better jobs for a higher salary so their lives and those of their children would be better than what they had known. And although the marriage was often stormy, I do believe, through it all, they never stopped loving each other.

Look at what they have now. For my mother, twenty years of Alzheimer's has meant not even being able to see her youngest child grow into an adult or even know her grandchildren. Her last ten years have been spent in a nursing home, alone. For my father, well, he's alone, with his wife in a nursing home in a near-vegetative state. No grand travel trips after retirement, no adventures as a couple after the kids are gone. There are no savings. My father's afraid to take long trips because they could call him home at any moment. The state now owns my mother's half of the house to cover the costs of her nursing home care, which was not covered by her retirement funds and her Social Security benefits. Most people don't realize that Medicare does not cover nursing home or in-home care for Alzheimer's patients. And nursing homes cost anywhere from $3,000 to sometimes $8,000 per month. Who can afford that while living on a pension?

For ten years my father cared for her at home. All extras—modifications to the house, hiring in-home care aides just to be able to go to the grocery store or have a day or weekend off—were all paid for out of pocket, slowly depleting their savings. My father's pension is reduced because he took early retirement at age fifty-five to care for Mother. So if he sells the house, the state gets half the proceeds; if he dies before Mother, the state gets the house and *all* the proceeds. He's trapped, just as my mother is trapped.

My mother decided to die on March 23, 1997, and it took twelve days for her body to catch up to her mind's intent. She stopped taking anything by mouth, refusing even water. This was no case of choking on food or having difficulty swallowing or "forgetting" how to eat and drink. She simply would not let anything pass through her lips ever again, choosing to end what nature kept sustaining.

I have no doubt that this was a deliberate choice on her part. During the days and nights I sat by her side, I watched her make that choice again and again. As they tried to brush her teeth, I saw her clamp her teeth shut with substantial force, fighting even that intrusion into her mouth. This included the little water-soaked sponges on a stick that were used to swab her teeth, gums, and tongue which were severely dehydrated and dry.

Billie was always conscious while this was happening. In fact, she was awake with her eyes open far more than I ever saw her sleeping. I detected some level of cognition throughout my stay with her. When I read to her from a book or magazine, she seemed to know I was reading to her. When I told her she would die soon and go to heaven, two tears slid down her cheeks—she had very little fluid in her body by then. When I got up to leave the room for any reason, her eyes would follow me. She never fell into a coma, even at the end. The night before she died, she never slept at all, and by this time she had been given a morphine shot and a seventy-two-hour morphine patch. Mother died when she simply did not take another breath.

Watching her fight to die, I found myself thinking about her quiet strength. My mother showed great determination and courage; I am glad that she was able to choose her own time to leave. She died on April 3, 1997, shortly after noon with my sister and a priest by her side, as she willed it.

During the terrible years, Carol's anger and sense of injustice for her mother's condition tore at her soul, but it also motivated her to look for answers to life's toughest questions: Why is this happening? Why was she allowed to suffer? What's fair about the wasted years? What about the smudged years?

Realistically, of course, we all have wasted years, hours of indolent nothingness, months of lethargic waste, years in which we accomplish little. These are truly wasted years of our own making. Billie's were wasted and smudged through no fault of her own.

In a beautiful eulogy to her mother, Carol talked about how her own personal quest to understand Alzheimer's had resolved itself into a kind of peace. "I've come to cherish those pieces of her that are within me," Carol says, "and I carry them forward, in my own way, with great pride and even greater love."

A Grim Slice of Alzheimer's

> *The mind is its own place, and in itself*
> *can make a Heaven of Hell, a Hell of Heaven.*
> —John Milton, *Paradise Lost*

Some demented persons become verbally abusive and others become controlled by the tangled, gnarled mess of the brain. The truth of the matter is that there are times when a family is in danger and the patient is dangerous. You are about to encounter the dark side of Alzheimer's no one likes to discuss. Unlike many Alzheimer's stories, this one scratches the monster's skin, and the fire comes from its most hateful moments. It is not a pretty story, but it resolves into an emotional moment when two people meet each other, simply and lovingly. Happily, this story happens less often today than it did even five years ago. As we develop even better techniques and medications to prevent such behavior, it will happen less frequently. This is why we support research. This is why we pray for the cure.

Geri Hall says there should be no violent stage. People with Alzheimer's become violent for several reasons:

- They are in pain or delirious. In this case, a doctor should be consulted.
- They are overwhelmed with fatigue, sensory input, too much change, and/or too many demands.
- They have a lifelong history of violence and know of no other way of coping.
- They become psychotic due to depressions, missed perceptions, or an atypical presentation of dementia.

All of the above can be treated except for the lifelong history. The most common reason for aggressive behavior is the fatigue factor. When this happens the violence is relieved by a slow, consistent routine with decreasing amounts of stimuli. Medications are only used very, very sparingly.

What's it like to be the daughter of an abusive, angry father whose life is a classic example of lifelong violence but who needs your care in his Alzheimer's years? When her father began to fail, Cathy did not hesitate to help the abuser and tormenter of her childhood. Cathy's dad was a big man, 225 pounds and muscular. A band of steel gray hair ringed his head. He had fair skin that tanned easily, blue eyes with bushy eyebrows. His kids were afraid of him. Born in 1911, he was raised to be "the man in the family." His siblings were girls, so as the only son his was a "no cry" world:

I wish I could say my father was a wonderful, loving man, but that was not the case. He was a bully, a know-it-all, and an arrogant person, a no-nonsense guy with little sense of humor. He was a man's man, a heavy smoker and drinker, tough, and more at home at sea than with the social and family skills that life on land demanded.

Cathy's mother led a seriously stormy life married to this man. His drinking was a major problem, causing them to lose friends. More than once she had to pull him out of a flophouse to get him back to his job as a captain in the United States Merchant Marines:

> I don't remember much about my childhood. Dad didn't know much about how to be a parent. He treated us kids as if we were the crew of his ship. He was a strict disciplinarian who never believed us. If we were telling the truth, we were punished because he thought we were lying. If we were caught in a lie, we were disciplined. If we cried when we were punished, he would punish us even harder saying, "I'll give you something to cry about."
>
> No matter how hard we tried to please him, it was never enough. What was the punishment? He would rant and rave, shout and holler, tell us that he wished we'd never been born, that he hated us, that we'd never amount to anything, that nobody would like us. He would threaten to throw us out of the house, threaten to send us to reform school, snarl, and be generally obnoxious. He would degrade us until we had not one iota of self-esteem left.
>
> When he was home it was no humor, no space, no slack. He was my father, but he wasn't my daddy until he went into the depths of Alzheimer's. It was then that he became the lovable little boy that I'm sure he was as a child. I think his abusive nature was a combination of his own insecurity, his own upbringing, and his career, but I wonder if our family will EVER be put together. The siblings cannot forget these early experiences. We are molded from a young age.

Recent research suggests that Alzheimer's can begin doing its damage even twenty to forty years before we actually see it in full bloom. Think of the possible changes in family life that early detection and treatment could bring to families like Cathy's. She says:

> In retrospect, the first sign of Dad's Alzheimer's appeared when he retired from the service very abruptly without talking to my

mom. That was about eighteen years before he died or about age sixty-two. After that, he would start household projects and never finish them or lose interest. In the early years, he had a big thing about household security—someone had to be at home at ALL times. Once he made Mom cancel her doctor's appointment because he and his friend were going for a walk. He just would not hear of leaving the house without security.

Alzheimer's had been in his family; his mother had been "very forgetful," and her brother had what was referred to as "extreme senility." And my uncle's son was also diagnosed with Alzheimer's.

Even with this family background, at the time Dad was diagnosed we had no idea what Alzheimer's was all about. We didn't know what we were dealing with, and so how could we know how to handle the problems? When we kept asking the doctor what was wrong with Dad, he just said that he was getting old. It was not long before I realized that we should not leave Dad alone. The doctor said nothing until about a year later. If we had known sooner, we would have been able to prepare for what was coming.

In the early stages, Dad would seem perfectly normal, but you just couldn't reason with him. For example, he would turn the thermostat up to eighty degrees because he was cold. Then the radiators got too hot, and he would panic. All the windows would be flung open with the radiators going full blast. It didn't matter how often we explained, he just didn't get it.

As the disease advanced, things got worse. Imagine seeing your father urinating indiscriminately around the house—like a dog or cat placing their scent—and ruining the rugs. I even found him urinating in the kitchen sink. On another occasion he started to play with the stove, almost causing a fire. That's when Mother really began to worry. He was falling a lot. Eventually, he couldn't dress or undress himself. He couldn't, or wouldn't, bathe or shave himself either, and obviously he couldn't be left alone. The stress began to build. I would take over at night when I got home, but it wasn't enough.

While taking care of him one day, the unthinkable occurred. At the very least it was an assault; at the worst, it was attempted rape. I was slapped around, thrown to the floor, with him groping me and trying to get my pants off. I knew he probably wouldn't get through the pants since he was already having trouble with buttons and zippers. I was completely unnerved, but I tried to keep my head. I didn't want him hurt, but I didn't want to get hurt either. It was important that he not get any angrier than he was. I really felt that my life was in danger.

Finally, I was able to get away and I just kept my distance. He tried to catch me, but when he did reach me, he couldn't remember why he was chasing me. The incident was over, and he had no memory of it at all. It scared the daylights out of me, and I hate to think about what it has done to my long-term mental health.

What about seeing your dad in a Geri chair with nothing on but a diaper? What about seeing him shuffling down the nursing home corridor with his pants down around his ankles, pooping as he goes along? What about taking him down to the garden in the nursing home, and as he steps off the elevator, he whips out his penis and just merrily pees away? A little old lady in a wheelchair said, "That's the ugliest thing I've ever seen!" Funny story now, but not so funny at the time.

And then it happened. I was visiting my father one day. He sat in his wheelchair and I was in a chair facing him. I had my feet hooked around the front wheels of his chair and was gently rubbing his arms and chest and talking to him. He looked me in the eye and said, "You're so nice, would you be my friend?" I started to cry. That statement meant two things to me: first, he didn't know me at that moment and second, being told that he wanted this "stranger" to be his friend in effect reversed part of the damage done in the terrible childhood years. I told him, "I'm already your friend, I'm your daughter."

A while later, in that same visit, he said to me, "You turned out good. Tell the others that I'm sorry." After a lifetime of criticism and abuse it broke my heart. But for that moment he did know who I was and he did remember. I still cry when I think of this visit.

I can't end this story without repeating. Violence is NOT normal in Alzheimer's. If it occurs, seek help immediately.

TWELVE
Faith, Hope, and Love

Few couples caught in the golden gleam of young love consider the possibility of a future marred by Alzheimer's. Love wraps us in a warm blanket of emotion, and we drift along letting the snug, half-remembered days of jobs and children carry us forward, happy, contented, and sure that it will always be so.

Then one day, one partner forgets to remember. She startles her mate with fits of anger. She forgets to turn off burners or is unable to find her way home when left to her own devices. Alzheimer's, Pick's Disease, Myocardial Infarction, whatever the diagnosis, the outcome is the same: watching the disintegration of the sum and substance of the one you love.

It is easy to love the lovable and chat with the reasonable. We parrot the words "for better or worse," our youth shielding us from what deep commitment this promise may hold. Alzheimer's puts our vows to the toughest test. For just as one partner is stricken by the disease, the other one loses his or her freedom and must care for this person he or she no longer knows. Their "happily ever after" is gone forever.

World's Greatest Pancake-maker

Bud Haltom voices his sense of loss in the poem written about his wife of fifty years:

Alzheimer's

How young and beautiful she was
Fortunate I was to win her hand
A full rewarding life was hers
But then by twist of fate, the weft
Did somehow shred and tatter
Loose ends blowing in the wind

Gone are the games of mental finesse
Gone are the jumbles and scrabble
Gone her creations of gourmet delight
Gone are the judgments and subtle charm

Her restless animation doth mock the lost ambition
And shattered goals lost logic can never more retrieve
The fury of my hell has not yet reached its peak
Say predictions and prognosis for the one I hold most dear

I remember when I specified
For traveling wave tubes built for space.
Satellites must only gradually lose their power.
"It must fail gracefully," I wrote
And never thought that God would ever
Request it for a mind or soul.
To aid in their replacement in an expeditious way.
—A. G. Holtum

Bud understood that to allow the love of his life to fail gracefully, his personal sacrifice would be great. Grace, in Alzheimer's, comes at great cost, but Bud's protective center would not let him allow Betty, his wife of fifty years, to die without dignity, without grace. This was his love.

At seventy-nine, Bud was quick to remind us that he was not yet eighty. He lived in Roswell, Georgia and was a true Renaissance man. His business card read "Scientist, Poet, Musician, and World's Greatest Pancake-maker. Specialty: electrodynamics, antennas, and waveguides." His white beard and bright smile left little doubt as to why he was asked to play Santa at local events.

Bud talked very little about his suffering; instead he talked about his wife, his family, about hope, faith, and his involvement in life:

Denial by the victim, as well as the loved ones, sometimes postpones the realistic and harsh diagnosis that must finally be confronted. After all, doesn't everyone have trouble keeping track of their car keys? We used to joke about how it wasn't much of a problem after duplicating and collecting six or seven sets. And women "always seem to misplace their purses," don't they?

Early on, Betty would sometimes wake up in the middle of the night crying. She said there was something happening in her brain

that was frightening, and she couldn't explain it. She had also suffered from what we thought were migraine headaches, so it was
back to another neurologist for a thorough physical examination.
The EEG was normal we were told, but X-rays indicated some
early signs of plaque build-up in some regions of the brain. This
could be a harbinger of dementia.

The mere suggestion of dementia triggered the angered emotional
response to "kill the messenger," and Betty suggested this young
doctor probably didn't know what he was talking about. About a
year later, when another neurologist ran a series of tests that resulted
in a definite diagnosis (as definite as possible without an autopsy), I
realized the most devastating aspect of Alzheimer's is that it is like
watching an unrelenting monster consume your loved one one small
bit at a time. Facing and confronting this reality, I believe, was my
lowest point. There is no defense and no retreat.

We had been married in February of 1941—not the best plan-
ning in the world. We had had six children, a miscarriage, and a
"preemie" who lived only a few hours. Betty had always been the
picture of health and looked at least ten years younger than her
chronological age. She could beat me at ping-pong as well as Scrabble. So full of energy, we were sure she would outlive me by many
years.

Betty had always taken care of our finances, opening checking and
savings accounts, paying bills, and the like. She began to ignore these
things, and I was determined to get her back in the swing of these activities so she could take charge in the event of my death. One of my
most disappointing moments took place when I realized this would
never happen. When I sat down with her at the dining room table
with the collection of mail and bills, she would invariably express the
desire to procrastinate. "Let's do it later," she would say. Her thoughtful moods became shorter and shorter, along with her attention span.
She would say, "You shouldn't have married me. I'm too simple for
you, not smart enough. We have so little in common." In a vain at-
tempt to add some humor to the conversation, I would say, "What
do you mean, not smart enough? You were smart enough to marry
me, weren't you?"

One day she came home from her hairdresser looking distraught.
She handed me the keys to her car and said, "I'm not driving in the
awful traffic anymore. It's too much. Next time I go, you can drop
me off." Then the next time came, I dropped her off and waited for

her phone call. It didn't come. When the shop told me she had left about an hour earlier, I got into my car and drove to town looking for her. Before long I spotted her. She said she had decided to walk home (a distance of about five miles).

A few years later came the irrational times. She would take her toothbrush from me and hold it under the water until the paste was gone or start to brush the basin. If I tried to guide her hand to her mouth, she would blaze with anger. Sometimes with her mouth full of toothpaste, water, and saliva, she would walk into the bedroom with cheeks bulging. I had to be careful at this point; sometimes she spit it out on the bed.

We usually awakened with the rising sun. I would think to myself, "Is the bed dry? Did the Depends do their job?" The night before had been another *drenching* experience, both outside and in the bed. I now have the extra-absorbent Depends.

"Want to go to the bathroom?" I ask.

"No," she answers. "I don't have to!"

"Yeah, yeah!" She walks into the bathroom and looks in the mirror.

"Turn to the right, dear, through the door to the toilet. See it?"

"No." I walk into the bathroom, turn her to the right, and gently guide her to the toilet.

"Oh, okay, okay. What now?"

"Just sit down, now, okay?"

"Is that all right, your majesty?"

"That's fine. I love you."

"How long does it take?"

I change the bed, gather the dirty clothes into a pile, and try to straighten the room a little. I hear water running in the toilet, and she says, "Is it all . . . what is she . . . Is that all?"

"Are you done dear?"

"Yes."

"Let's go wash our hands now." I lead her to the sink and hand her the soap. She puts some on her hands and makes a lather. "Let's rinse now," I say. Sometimes she would hold the soap in one hand, not seeming to understand to rub them together. Then I had to wash her hands for her."

"Okay! Okay!"

"Let's get dressed now." I change the pad on her Depends and hand her a clean bra and panties. In her bra and panties she starts to make the bed, and I am amazed at how well she performs this chore, so I step back and watch. I must not leave the room at this point, because if I do I would come back to find she had put on two or three more pairs of panties, two or three blouses, and two or three more pairs of slacks, one on top of the other.

A few years later, things really began to fall apart.

That night was truly traumatic. We watched TV until about 8:30 and suddenly Betty seemed to freeze in a slouched-over position and couldn't even walk without a lot of help. I thought of my younger days when I could carry her without too much difficulty. Unfortunately, I'm too old to do that anymore. Needless to say, it took me about half an hour to get her up the stairs, and I had visions of having to install a cart and rail. There is a name for such an apparatus, but I can't think of it.

When I told the doctor, he suggested we put her in the hospital and warned me that we had better make arrangements for a nursing home because things are going to get a lot worse. However, after making all the arrangements to admit her to the hospital, I noticed Betty was becoming more mobile and alert, so we temporarily called things off. Alzheimer's can sometimes play hide-and-seek with you. Friday, we all were surprised when Paul, our son, flew in from California on a business trip and took two days off to visit us. You should have seen Betty's face. She was so happy to see her youngest and really enjoyed his visit.

About six weeks later, I thought Betty was having a stroke, at first, when she was unable to climb the stairs. Ellen, my nurse-daughter, called the doctor and they admitted her to the geriatric center. Her wandering and present condition caused the doctor to recommend she be admitted to a nursing home. There were no beds available until Faith and Ellen made a last-minute plea to the Presbyterian Village.

Our son, Ed, who is the star singer and musician in the family, was visiting us at the time, so the director of the home arranged for us to have a jam session and cut a videotape while we were entertaining the patients. This led to a regular routine of entertaining the patients both on the guitar and piano and was a big boost to my morale.

During the next two and a half years, Betty was a resident of the village. I visited her about three times a week and later began to play the hymns every Sunday morning for the special Sunday School class. I got to know all thirty-seven patients in the Alzheimer's unit by their first names and became an official volunteer. My main function was entertainment with old songs that were miraculously still imbedded in the memories of these residents. And, oh yes! At Christmas, I also played the role of Santa!

But beneath all the jollity and activity was a man watching his love disappear. His sparkling eyes belied the pain that he was feeling. This he expressed in his poetry:

The Alzheimer's Enigma

How quietly she sits and stares.
Her feet do not respond
to instructions from her brain
and sometimes shake while resting
on the props of her wheelchair.
The spoon she holds does not move
while her gracious, patient, caregiver
feeds her with firm and steady hand.
What is in her thoughts and mind,
as her eyes widen when she sees me,
her lover and companion for over fifty years?
Perceptual and conceptual prowess
are vanquished as aphasia grows.
Incarcerated in a living tomb,
she now seems passive and content.
The pain endured for these last years,
is not gone, it now resides
in those who love her dearly.
"Do not take my loved one, please!"
I prayed to God so fervently,
Never dreaming compromise
and losing her so gradually.

—A. G. Holtum

During this time, Betty began to lose mobility and her aphasia[1] was increasing. Wheelchair-bound and talking less and less, she never lost the ability to recognize me or her children as well as some of her grandchildren. She was always glad to see me, and I could always make her laugh and smile.

How I miss the person she used to be, but I learned to love the person she was and always looked forward to seeing her. The cynical side of her personality was now waning, and she exhibited a lovable nature that was readily recognized by those around her, including the staff and other residents. During our visits, I would hold her hands in mine and tell her all the things that were going on with our large family, including the birth of each new great-grandchild. I did all the talking, and I really did not know if she understood what I was saying, but I always assumed she did from the look of satisfaction I read in her soft brown eyes. On the days I entertained the residents on the guitar or piano, she would sit alongside me in her wheelchair.

One Sunday, after I had played the hymns and visited her as usual, one of my nurse-daughters called me late that night and told me the staff had called her to say that Betty had suffered a stroke and was at the county hospital. Both my daughters and I visited her during the wee hours Monday morning. Betty was comatose and remained in a coma until she died less than twenty-four hours later.

My dear sweet wife of over fifty-four years was gone. I spent days looking through the pictures of our life together, but looking at them brought tears. My daughters and one of my grandchildren stayed with me while I made funeral arrangements that I should have planned much earlier. All of my children and nine of our grandchildren came to the funeral. What a comfort my big family was during this trauma. Members of the family composed some poetry for the service and our older son recorded some hymns on a tape that was played.

I continue to dream about Betty. I see her and touch her, hugging her and kissing her in images that are vivid and real. Inevitably the unwanted logic imbedded in my rational mind would summon up the conflicts that would cause her to vanish and I would awaken with my hands grasping my pillow and tears in my eyes.

It's hard not to be reminded of all the good times. At night I see her picture and ask her to visit me in my dreams. When I leave in the car, it doesn't seem right that she's not there beside me. When I shop for groceries, I dream of her walking down the aisle with me. But then I am roused from my wishful fantasy by the stark, cruel realization that she is gone from my real world forever. Forever.

When I look back, I realize that in spite of the loss and trauma that confronted me, I have had multiple blessings. Consider all the exciting and stimulating events and activities in my large and close-knit family, without which I could have easily descended into deep despair. I believe that I have learned that one of the secrets of life and living is interaction with those around us and the free exchange of real concern and love.

As Paul said, "Of faith, hope, and love, the greatest of these is love."
A. G. Holtum joined his wife Betty two years ago.

Mourning Dove: The Alzheimer's Divorce

> *I stood on tiptoe gazing into the distance*
> *Interminably gazing at the road*
> *that had taken you.*
> —Wife of Ch'in Chia

Bud's story is an example of a man's tender caring for a woman he has loved for over fifty years. John and Sarah have been married about forty years and are about to be divorced. This is not the legal divorce of two people who are finished with one another; this is a divorce occasioned by dementia.

John was stricken about eleven years ago with what the doctors have diagnosed as vascular dementia or multi-infarct dementia. Although the causes are different, MID and Alzheimer's have some similarities. MID is caused by small strokes and can plateau for a period and then worsen upon the occasion of another stroke. Alzheimer's has a more gradual and steady downward spiral. With her spouse mentally absent, Sarah believes she has no choice but to walk her future path alone. Sarah and I are friends and I have her permission to share her letters with you.

> October 10, 1995
>
> I've gone through a great deal of agitation and verbally aggressive behavior on my husband's part, and I have sought assistance with my own anger and depression. There now is a sort of peace in this household. I find I no longer try to hold on to his previous level of functioning and can more readily accept his bizarre and declining episodes. I know John's sensory input is going. He has a kind of tunnel-like vision, a loss of smell (couldn't smell a recent forest fire), less taste sense (wants all food heavily seasoned), and difficulty making meaning out of sounds.

November 5, 1995

When I get to this point (needing a living will), I want to let nature take its course if I can. I even thought about refusing my husband's flu shot this year but decided I couldn't let go yet. Such hard and awful decisions to make.

November 7, 1995

My husband confuses me with someone else. The first time I was so surprised I cried, and then he realized what he had done. Several other times I tried to reorient him and the last time about six months ago, I asked him who I was. He said I was a wonderful friend and he would like to marry me. I shall always treasure that reply. It hasn't happened for a long time, and I'm sure I don't know if it's just because . . . or whether something was resolved.

How I wish we could avoid expressing frustration by yelling, but it is an easy thing to give into. Although my husband forgets why he was yelled at, he doesn't forget that he was yelled at. I try to apologize with a simple explanation, not that I think he understands, but it seems to convey to him that everything is okay.

John seems to have settled down, for the present anyway, but this week he keeps telling me I'm not nice to him. Sometimes I think I want to throw the wash water at him. He's very confused not knowing where to pee, where to get a tissue to blow his nose. He has tried several times to put his mittens on his feet and fights with Hamilton. I swear that cat knows he can get John mad, then he runs under the couch, and John is poised with a newspaper or shoe or whatever, and I'm not sure he won't hurt him. I can see the humor in the two of them. It would make a good TV show.

January 10, 1996

Sue, I cannot let him go if there is the least chance of him going on for a while longer. He isn't all I have, but he is most of my life, and placement in a home is so undeniably final. Then he will never come home again. There is no more hope. There is no more "us." I know this time will come, but I'm not quite ready for it yet. Not yet.

I think I really hope John will go to sleep and not wake up. Hard as that seems, I think that's better than struggling every waking moment to make sense of something in a world that isn't making sense. He gets in such a panic at those times. I just don't want John to struggle or be afraid. As for me, I hide my anger, but it's there, loud and clear. And I cry a lot. I just wish things were different.

January 22, 1996

John's language isn't so good. Sometimes there are no nouns at all and after finishing a sentence, he'll say, "That wasn't too good, was it?" We usually laugh and go on, but sometimes it makes him angry. So sometimes it's John I'm talking to and sometimes it isn't. That's one of the hardest things for me.

I find that our way of life before dementia has made things difficult. We were both independent, so in our marriage things were divided into my area, his area, and our area. When the darkness and the pit started to envelop us, it meant I had to start doing ALL areas. Even now it's very difficult for me to keep everything going.

I don't think I can say this illness has brought us closer. We *were* very close. We still have each other, but there's a space now. It seems to widen. He's no longer a husband or companion. This was the hardest thing I had to accept, and I almost lost both our lives before I did.

March 15, 1996

Oh, Sue. I can't stop crying. I've cried for two days. I honestly don't know what to do. I get no good sleep. He paces and paces and paces. Even though I try to keep my voice appropriate and non-threatening, he refuses to do anything. I tried videos, but he only watches for a minute or two. If I get impatient, he gets irritable. He follows me around, and even now I have to watch that he's not reading what I'm writing on the computer. He never wants a meal, but snack, snack, snack. Munching, always munching. It's really driving me crazy. I'm beginning to intensely dislike this man I'm living with.

My daughter and I visited an open house at a new nursing facility yesterday. What a loser. An outside area about 100′x100′, all plastic and locks. There was plenty of walking space, but no activity space at all. Price $145 per day. I think I'll choose the first home I see. This looking around is too emotionally draining.

Sarah decided to take a week of respite. She took John to the nursing home for the week—their first week apart in many years. When uneasiness about the separation persists this can be a good option. Many nursing homes and assisted-living facilities offer this temporary care.

April 16, 1996

I went to bed about nine with a book, read for about an hour and turned out the light. Well, I didn't sleep until around 3:30. Just all so different. Called the center, and they said he's had a wonderful day. A few times he couldn't find his room, that's all. They called this morning and said again how smooth things were going. I'm so glad he's not unhappy. That would break my heart even though I recognize this is a step.

April 21, 1996

Oh, what a week. Both a dismal failure and a rousing success. Can you guess in what order? I just couldn't handle it. I cried and cried and hardly slept. John, on the other hand, settled in very well, got upset when he saw in the paper about a fatal car crash and the picture of a car like mine, but with an explanation and another Haldol, all was well.

But he cried when I came this morning and has been pretty emotional today. We fell asleep on the couch this afternoon holding hands.

As her friend, I know that what Sarah leaves unsaid speaks volumes. She has finally accepted the fact that John has arrived at the point of separation. As she continues, you can see her way of saying goodbye to her husband:

April 23, 1996

Hi Sue! A good night's sleep and another day! Not so bleak today. We went for a walk to the river and found some birds' nests and trout lily sprouting, a few geese on their way home. It's days like this that let me feel I can bear this for a long time, but down under I know better. If only there were some consistency in this disease. We're both pretty mellow at the moment. John wants to be close, and I don't want to encourage his disorientation before I have to. The nursing center said that he is at an appropriate level to remain there, so we have tentatively made a plan for sometime in the next four months.

May 14, 1996

Called the Alzheimer's Center yesterday and found John is next on the list but with no assurance as to timing. I was pretty discouraged when I found the wet bed this morning, and I found he had used the wastebasket beside the toilet once during the day. Seems to have straightened out now for the time being. At least I have the bed well "proofed" now. Such an increase in restlessness and confusion, with just enough clarity thrown in to mix me up. In a way I was glad my older son was here to see the confusion because usually John gets in the "social mode" and performs quite well to the casual onlooker.

I even yelled at John this morning after NOTHING would keep him from putting used toilet paper in his shirt pocket. THEN he told me it was very serious to leave the milk on the counter, not in the refrigerator. We had a silent breakfast, and when I was dressing he brought in a Mother's Day card from the counter and said he wanted me to know what a nice person I was. Lord, the inconsistencies in this disease. How do I cope?

May 21, 1996

The residential center called and they have a bed available. I had the strongest feeling Sunday night that someone fell and broke a hip, they would call Monday, and John would go this week. That's what happened. Although I truly think this is for the best, what an empty-pit feeling. How I hate this disease! I don't WANT to start my life over again all alone! What a big empty house! And a broken heart. Why, dear God, WHY??

May 25, 1996 (The day Sarah placed John in a facility)

Hi Friend,

Yes this day is finished. It went smoothly enough but not great. It was incredibly difficult as everyone says. No angry agitation, just sadness. I'm afraid to call, afraid they'll say he's upset. I think I'd go get him if I heard that, so . . . until tomorrow.

August 2, 1996

Sue, I really don't know what I'm doing. I don't think I'm punishing myself, but I sure am unwell. I didn't sleep and didn't eat much for about a month after John's admission. My greatest desire is to curl up in my old worn-out velour recliner with the doors locked so no one can bother me. Yet I'm continuing to do what needs to be done. I've seen Jim (psychologist) and he tells me I'm a walking checklist for depression. Tells me to meditate daily, get exercise, leave the house everyday, and so forth. Sounds great but takes oh-so-much energy that I don't have. I'm taking Zoloft. My doctor describes it as "son of Prozac."

August 5, 1996

Today I'm doing better. Nausea has subsided and although I'm not very hungry, I'm eating better and getting a little sleep. My grandson was here for a while and he took my mind off the situation. But as soon as he left, I felt overwhelmingly sad. I can see that look on John's face that says I'm not really his wife anymore. It makes me cry. I guess our relationship is DEAD, DEAD, DEAD. He was so confused when I visited him today. It was too hot to go for a walk, so I packed some soda and fruit and bread and thought we'd drive to a spot and sit under a tree in the shade. He had none of his usual interest, but just wandered and wandered. So we stayed right at the home.

I'm tempted to go see him again tomorrow, but what good will it do? I'm feeling abandoned. I'm not sure if I can manage to get through all this. Question: Is the facility becoming his family and his home? Is there no place for me in it? What do I do then? I circle around and it always comes back to this. I don't know how people cope.

August 21,1996

We both had a bad visit today. I brought him home and could see he wasn't being held together by more than a frazzled string. When I took him back, he said he was going to walk home. The first resistance I've seen in three months, and I couldn't help but cry. Later, I heard from the nurse that he'd tried to choke another patient. An increase in his Haldol seemed to handle the problem, but this roller coaster is killing me.

February 9, 1997

I tried to be my analytical self today and compared John's appearance and walking behavior with some others. Not good. Then I did some of the tests they use for drug-related behavior. Unlikely. I brought him a Valentine's card and he couldn't open the envelope. He just wanted to sleep. My head says I need to let him go, get this thing done with, and be finished with the suffering. My heart says, "Don't go, John. Don't leave me yet!" The pit gets deeper. I know the reality of going on without John is getting closer, but I don't want it to. And it doesn't matter at all what I want.

More than five years have passed, John still lives on in a nursing facility, and Sarah is still waiting for the other shoe to drop. The past is not complete, and the future cannot yet begin. The strain on Sarah continues as she tries to fill her days with reading, volunteer work, and an occasional trip with friends. She concerns herself with mending and fixing needed repairs around her country home, and time passes. Her children are close and the grandchildren are there to give her love, but, alas, aside from a weekly visit to the nursing home, John is no longer a part of her life. This is the divorce that Alzheimer's causes.

I recently had a letter from Sarah:

What's it like to visit an empty shell with no acknowledgement whatsoever? The cruelest part is the failure to die, to avoid this ultimate insult to personal dignity.

Epilogue

*Philosophy is perfectly right in saying
that life must be understood backwards.
But then one forgets the other clause—
that it must be lived forward.*
—Soren Kierkegaard, *Journals and Papers*

The day I looked up, felt the breeze, and knew it was time to reconsider the future was the day I knew I had mended. I can remember the exact moment. With relief, I somehow knew I had completed my return journey. With Mother's illness our family had entered the depth of a great, long winter, but now, finally, we were able to look within ourselves and find the beginnings of what Albert Camus called "an invincible summer." The blackbirds were once again singing along the riverbank and I could feel the touch of joy one experiences at just being alive. My return journey had allowed me to once again discover the spring within myself.

The need to analyze one's actions is often seen as a liability, and yet there was no other path for me to follow. Those who make it a rule of thumb to never allow themselves to feel regret and to never look back are to be envied. Such persons would consider my actions an appalling waste of energy, and yet, for me, it has been an absolute necessity. How strong is our courage? How resolute is our endurance? How can one go forward into future times of joy and sorrow without understanding what exists within? Am I compassionate or careless? Am I distant or caring? Am I growing or am I stagnant? For me, self-knowledge is won at great cost and contemplation, and still, it remains a study in progress.

*What lies behind us and what lies before us are
small matters compared to what lies within us.*
—Ralph Waldo Emerson

In his or her own way, many of us engage in numerous return journeys during a lifetime. Obstacles, guilt, and grief are a part of life, and each struggle sharpens our strengths or it weakens and erodes our already tentative lease on our fragile self-worth. Without a personal evaluation we ricochet from one crisis to another, never investigating the healthy baggage we will need to confront the next difficulty. Recently a caregiver, in describing his view of Alzheimer's, simply said, "Failure." We understood exactly what he meant; there is no successful conclusion to Alzheimer's and caregivers are left empty-handed and empty-hearted, unsure of what they did and how they did it. When it's all over, most of us need to return to the scene and ask ourselves difficult questions and rediscover ourselves in the quicksand that's left behind.

In her book *Kitchen Table Wisdom*, Dr. Rachel Remen tells a Hindu story of how the god, Shiva, drops a bag of gold in front of a miserably poor man. The poor man steps over the bag of gold, thinking it is a rock. "I might have ruined my sandals," he says. And he goes on his way.

Remen continues:

> It seems that Life drops many bags of gold in our path. Rarely do they look like what they are. I asked my patient if Life has ever dropped him a bag of gold that he has recognized and used to enrich his life. He smiles at me, "Cancer," he says simply. "I thought you'd guess" (Remen 88–89).

My mother's Alzheimer's, as awful an experience as it was, helped me learn the first lesson of human existence: if we wish to be forgiving persons, we first need to forgive ourselves. I had a terrible time being compassionate toward myself for my caregiving failures. A friend of mine was kicking herself for giving her mother an over-the-counter medication during her final stages that we have since discovered may be contra-indicated for Alzheimer's patients. My friend knew no better. She must forgive herself. Personally I had to forgive myself for the lack of knowledge and empathy I felt I lacked, and I had to absolve myself of my guilt for those things left undone and those things which should not have been done.

For comfort, I look at the sky and tell Mother that someday she and I will meet and I will ask absolution for all past faux pas. Without my return journey I would still be stuffing my feelings of failure, grief, and guilt; I would be superficially engaged in life and yet lacking "something." I would not have recognized my "bag of gold."

I had always told my children that life isn't all laughter and games, yet I became angry and disbelieving when the time for weeping and reality came to me. During Mother's illness the thorns of actuality scratched my soul, but now I thank them for having taught me to be stronger. I know I can still be hurt—passionate humanity demands we honor this open wound—but I have learned skills necessary to surviving grief and pain: forgiveness, compassion, an open mind, and the ability to withhold judgment of others. Longfellow put it well when he wrote, "Let us then be up and doing, with a heart for any fate."

I have learned that each stage in life is important, the going out as well as the coming in, and I knew that my mother's final confused life had meaning. It changed my family in some very meaningful ways. We have always loved one another, but now there is just a touch more; we will be there when sad times come, we will cherish just a bit more, and we will take more time to look beyond the obvious to find one another. All is not found in the words we use—seeking to understand is all.

Being a compliant student, I always knew how important it was to have the answers, but I have learned that it is also important to know the questions. An eyes-open, questioning attitude is the catalyst for change in Alzheimer's care. Because a few leaders, along with thousands of intuitive caregivers on the front lines, have asked the question, "What kind of care do Alzheimer's patients need," many changes are evolving in our treatment of dementia. It isn't enough to have simple book knowledge, using information gained in training. It isn't enough to warehouse our loved ones and keep them from wandering. It certainly isn't enough to sit them in front of a TV set for hours.

Our questioning attitude has opened our eyes to the fact that Alzheimer's patients retain many skills and emotions, powerful avenues through which we can reach them and care for them. Activities, love, and a sense of humor are some of our greatest tools in making life meaningful for our loved ones. Adult day care centers are showing us the way with a day filled with creative activities. Unfortunately, many so-called Alzheimer's facilities have not yet made this turnaround and, because of staff restrictions, money crunches, and other excuses, we have only begun the battle. This is what we all want for our loved ones: an active, meaningful, dignified existence.

We must say to ourselves, as David Hyde Pierce recently said when appearing on TV for the Alzheimer's Association, "I never want to see another human being go through this again." Once our personal battle is waged we are duty-bound to join the struggle for extended research funds, more home care for Alzheimer's patients, and the physical, occupational, and speech therapies and mental health services open to victims of other diseases.

A Return Journey has also shown me that I did some things right. We all make many very difficult decisions along the Alzheimer's path and, all in all, I feel satisfied that generally those I had to make were for the best at that point in time. Placing Mother in a facility was the most difficult, guilt-wrenching decision I had ever made, but it was for the best. She had companionship and distractions outside herself. Luckily, this was an activities-rich environment and she knew she was among loving persons. Another thing I did that I still feel was right was to try not to make any decision for Mother that I wouldn't be willing for my children to make for me. Without fail, Alzheimer's caregivers loathe the decisions they are forced to make in caring for the loved one, but they, like me, come out of the pit knowing that they have done their best.

Now that Mother is gone we are left with memories and dreams, dreaming of the day when we corral this disease and extinguish its ability to hurt. Currently, I volunteer for the Alzheimer's Association and have served on the local helpline. I have helped with a support group and a strategy group and I support Alzheimer's research as much as I am financially able. This tells you what I am doing, but it doesn't tell you how I feel. As we have said before, time mends. It doesn't heal; it sews us up and pats us on the head. We still walk wounded, but just as a broken bone often grows stronger as it mends, many of us feel we are tougher for the hurt.

The joy of everyday things—my grandchildren's laughter and my children's love—has become more precious to me now than before I experienced this terrible disease. I try to hear the birds sing and to be thankful for my blessings. I peek at my dear husband when he doesn't know I'm watching and cherish the years we have left to share. I pray for his health and am trying to be more diligent in caring for my own. I will continue to be deeply involved in my life, always searching for the deepest eddies and looking for answers that I just know are hidden somewhere waiting to be found.

It is my hope that those of us who have stared this disease in the face will increase our vigilance and creative response to the challenge. It will require that we dirty our hands and engage in the soul-searching work of supporting creative research and on-the-edge care for the victims of dementia. Making *A Return Journey* into our uncertainty and doubt about current practices can, perhaps, lead us to better care for those we love and to unexpected riches for ourselves. God bless us all.

> *. . . when the fight begins within himself,*
> *A man's worth something.*
> —Robert Browning

Let us then "be up and doing."

Notes

ONE. *The Enormity of It All*

1. Early-onset Alzheimer's: when a person is diagnosed before the ages of sixty to sixty-five.
2. Medicaid: a program jointly funded by each state and the federal government that provides medical aid for those who fall below a certain income level.

FOUR. *Developing a Caregiver's Mindset*

1. Morris, along with another Alzheimer's-diagnosed person, submitted a paper to the plenary session of the Australian Association at the end of March 2001.
2. "Memories in the Making" program: a program sponsored by the Alzheimer's Association that encourages art in the lives of Alzheimer's patients.

FIVE. *Day by Day with the Stranger*

1. Power of Attorney (POA): legal document, usually called a Durable Power of Attorney (DPOA), that allows one to act in another's behalf.
2. Safe Return: a national program that provides bracelets or dog tags to identify Alzheimer's wanderers. For more information call or visit your local Alzheimer's Association office or visit www.alz.org.

SIX. *A Few Extra Moments, Please*

1. Business card-sized information cards available through your local Alzheimer's Association office.

NINE. *With Every Goodbye We Learn*

1. Hospice: originally a shelter or lodging, we now know is as a sheltering group—nurses, social workers, etc.—who care for the dying.
Sometimes this is done in another facility and often it is done at home. Today we consider calling in hospice services if our loved one has less than six months to live. This is, of course, only a general rule.

TWELVE. *Faith, Hope, and Love*

1. Aphasia: an inability to articulate ideas.

Appendix A

Understanding Stages and Symptoms of Alzheimer's Disease

Common Changes in Mild Alzheimer's Disease:

- Loses spark or zest for life—does not start anything
- Loses recent memory without a change in appearance or casual conversation
- Loses judgment about money
- Has difficulty with new learning and making new memories
- May stop talking to avoid making mistakes
- Has shorter attention span and less motivation to stay with an activity
- Easily loses way going to familiar places
- Resists change or new things
- Has trouble organizing and thinking logically
- Asks repetitive questions
- Withdraws, loses interest, is irritable, is not as sensitive to others' feelings, is uncharacteristically angry when frustrated or tired
- Won't make decisions. For example, when asked what she wants to eat, says, "I'll take what she is having."
- Takes longer to do routine chores and becomes upset if rushed or if something unexpected happens
- Forgets to pay, pays too much, or forgets how to pay; may hand the checkout person a wallet instead of the correct amount of money
- Forgets to eat, eats only one kind of food, or eats constantly
- Loses or misplaces things by hiding them in odd places or forgets where things go, such as putting clothes in the dishwasher

Common Changes in Moderate Alzheimer's Disease:

- Changes in behavior, concern for appearance, hygiene, and sleep become more noticeable
- Mixes up identity of people, such as thinking a son is a brother or a wife is a stranger
- Poor judgment, creates safety issues when left alone; may wander or risk exposure, poisoning, falls, self-neglect, or exploitation
- Has trouble recognizing familiar people and own objects; may take things that belong to others
- Continuously repeats stories, favorite words, statements, or motions like tearing tissues
- Has restless, repetitive movements in late afternoon or evening like pacing, trying doorknobs, fingering draperies
- Cannot organize thoughts or follow logical explanations
- Has trouble following written notes or completing tasks
- Makes up stories to fill in gaps in memory. For example, might say, "Mama will come for me when she gets off work."
- May be able to read but cannot formulate the correct response to a written request
- May accuse, threaten, curse, fidget, or behave inappropriately, such as kicking, hitting, biting, screaming, or grabbing
- May become sloppy or forget manners
- May see, hear, smell, or taste things that are not there
- May accuse spouse of an affair or family members of stealing
- Naps frequently or awakens at night believing it is time to go to work
- Has more difficulty positioning the body to use the toilet or sit in a chair
- May think mirror image is following him or television story is happening to her
- Needs help finding the toilet, using the shower, remembering to dress, and dressing for the weather or occasion
- Exhibits inappropriate sexual behavior, such as mistaking another individual for a spouse. Forgets what is private behavior, and may disrobe or masturbate in public.

Common Changes in Severe Alzheimer's:

- Doesn't recognize self or close family
- Speaks in gibberish, is mute, or is difficult to understand
- May refuse to eat, chokes, or forgets to swallow
- May repetitively cry out, pat, or touch everything
- Loses control of bowel and bladder
- Loses weight and skin becomes thin and tears easily
- May look uncomfortable or cry out when transferred or touched
- May have seizures, frequent infections, falls
- May sleep more
- Needs total assistance for all activities of daily living

* Adapted from: Gwyther, Lisa P. *Caring for People with Alzheimer's Disease: A Manuel for Facility Staff.* 2d. ed. Washington, D.C.: American Health Care Association, 2001.

Appendix B

Caregiver's Self-rating Scale

Below is a scale to evaluate your level of caregiving. It has been adapted from an article in "Co-op Networker; Caregiver of Older Persons" by Judy Bradley. It is an excellent effort to provide some guidelines for caregivers and to evaluate your level of care and value which you give your care-receiver and yourself.

The scale is a 1–10 continuum that describes the various styles of caring. Circle the number or numbers which best describes your level of care.

1   2   3   4   5   6   7   8   9   10

1. Abandonment: to withdraw protection or support or to actively abuse your care-receiver

2. Neglect: to allow life-threatening situations to persist or to display consistent coldness or anger

3. Detachment/Aloofness: to maintain an air of detachment or being aloof, perfunctory in your care, no genuine concern, only obligation; concerned only with physical well-being of your care-receiver

4. General Support: given freely, with a guarded degree of warmth and respect, occasional feelings of manipulation; concerned with both emotional and physical well-being of care-receiver

5. Expressed empathy: the ability to feel what your care-receiver feels; a quality relationship where feelings can be freely expressed and are received with non-judgmental positive regard

6. Sympathy: feeling sorry for care-receiver, giving sympathy, focusing on the losses experience by care-receiver

7. Occasional over-involvement: care characterized by periodic attempts to "do for" rather than "be with"

8. Consistent over-involvement: care-receiver regarded as object of series of tasks which must be performed

9. Heroic over-involvement: care characterized by sometimes frantic and desperate attempts to provide for every possible need your care-receiver has; increased dependence, care-receiver not allowed independence

10. Fusion of personalities: between caregiver and care-receiver; the caregiver's needs no longer have any value of meaning; the caregiver has abandoned him/herself to needs of the care-receiver

You can place yourself on the scale of caregiving to determine how you value your care-receiver as compared to yourself. The low numbers (1, 2, 3) give little or no value (honor) to the needs of your care-receiver. The high numbers (8, 9, 10) give little or no value to your own needs. The numbers in the middle (4, 5, 6, 7) are where you will find a balance between undercare and overcare. Neither of the two extremes is healthy. They represent positions where you are not helping your care-receiver.

Appendix C

Caregiver Stress Test

The following test will help you become aware of your feelings, pressures, and stress you currently feel:

	Seldom	Sometimes	Often	Usually
I find I can't get enough rest				
I don't have enough time for myself				
I don't have time to be with other family members besides the person I care for				
I feel guilty about my situation				
I don't get out much anymore				
I have conflict with the person I care for				
I cry every day				
I worry about having enough money to make ends meet				
I don't feel I have enough knowledge or experience to give care as well as I'd like				

If the response to one or more of these areas is "usually true" or "often true" it may be time to begin looking for help with caring for the care-receiver and help in taking care of yourself.

*From: Torres-Stanovik, Robert, ed. *The Caregiver's Handbook*. The Caregiver Education and Support Services, Seniors Counseling and Training, Case Management Services of the San Diego County Mental Health Association, Online, 1990. <http://www.adrc.wustl.edu/alzheimer/care.html>

Appendix D

Ten Ways to Help a Family Dealing with Alzheimer's Disease

Friends are an important source of support for an Alzheimer family. Even if they live far away, there's still plenty you can do. Here are ten easy ways to help:

1. Keep in touch. Call, send a card, visit. Continue to keep in touch even if you don't get a response. It's a simple yet important way to show you care.

2. Do little things—they mean a lot: when cooking, make extra portions and drop off a meal in a freezable and disposable container.

3. Give them a break. Everyone needs a little time for himself or herself. Offer to stay with the Alzheimer person so family members can run errands. Offer to take the Alzheimer person to lunch so the family can enjoy a quiet minute at home.

4. Be specific when offering assistance. Caregivers find it hard to ask for help. Give specific suggestions of things you are willing to do—shovel the walkways, mow the lawn, grocery shop, fix the plumbing.

5. Be alert. Learn about Alzheimer's and how it impacts the family. Know how to recognize a problem and respond to common behaviors such as wandering.

6. Provide a change of scenery. Plan an activity that includes the entire family. Be sure to include the person with Alzheimer's if the caregiver feels it is appropriate.

7. Learn to listen. Sometimes those affected by Alzheimer's just need to talk with someone. You don't need to provide answers—just be a compassionate listener. Try not to question or judge, but rather, support and accept.

8. Care for the caregiver. Encourage caregivers to take care of themselves. Pass along useful information and offer to attend a support group with them.

9. Remember all family members. The person with Alzheimer's will appreciate your visit even if he or she is unable to show it. Be attentive to the needs of all family members.

10. Get involved. Make a contribution to your local Alzheimer's Association or volunteer your time at the local chapter. Your involvement tells your friend that you care.

*Alzheimer's Association of Orange County. *Ten Ways to Help a Family Dealing with Alzheimer's Disease.* Alzheimer's Association of Orange County, Online, 20 June 2003. <http://www.alzoc.org/support/Helplinetopics/CG_10ways.htm>

Resources

Alzheimer's Association. "Alzheimer's Challenges Couples' Closest Ties." *Alzheimer's Association National Newsletter* 13, 2 (summer 1995).

Alzheimer's Association. "Caring Across the Miles." *Advances* 19, 3 (fall 1999).

Alzheimer's Association. *Facts: About Alzheimer's Disease* (PR6172). Alzheimer's Association, Pamphlet, 2002.

Alzheimer's Association. "General Statistics/Demographics." Alzheimer's Association, Online, 02 January 2003.
<http://www.alz.org/AboutAD/Statistics.htm>

Alzheimer's Association. *Living with Early-Onset Alzheimer's Disease* (ED2062). Alzheimer's Association, Pamphlet, 1999.

Alzheimer's Association. *Overview of Alzheimer's Disease and Related Disorders* (ED2052). Alzheimer's Association, Pamphlet, 1997.

Alzheimer's Association. "Survey Finds Large Communication Gap Between Doctors and Alzheimer's Caregivers." Alzheimer's Association, Online, 07 June 2001.
<http://www.alz.org/Media/newsreleases/archived/060601alzsurvey.html>

Alzheimer's Association. *Statistics: About Alzheimer's Disease* (LIB620Z). Alzheimer's Association, Pamphlet, 2002.

Alzheimer's Association. Thinking Outside the Box: "An Alternative Approach to Care, a Feature on Thinking Outside the Box." *Advances* 19, 2 (summer 1999).

Alzheimer's Disease and Related Disorders Association, Inc. *Steps to Getting a Diagnosis.* Alzheimer's Disease and Related Disorders Association, Inc., Pamphlet, 1996.

Aplin, Cary T., M.A. "Group Therapy for Family Caregivers of Patients with Alzheimer's Disease." *Awareness* (fall 1996).

Austin, James H., M.D. *Zen and the Brain: Toward an Understanding of Meditation and Consciousness.* Cambridge: MIT Press, 1999.

Barrett, William. *Irrational Man.* New York: Doubleday, 1962.

Bell, Virginia and David Troxel. *The Best Friends Approach to Alzheimer's Care.* Baltimore: Health Professions Press, 1997.

Cowley, Geoffrey, with Anne Underwood. "Alzheimer's: Unlocking the Mystery." *Newsweek,* Online, 31 January 2000. <http://archives.newsbank.com>

CNN. com. "Is Stress Taking a Toll on Your Health?" CNN Your Health, Online transcript, 30 December 2000. <http://www.cnn.com/TRANSCRIPTS.html>

Dempsey, Marge and Sylvia Baago. "Latent Grief: the Unique and Hidden Grief of Carers of Loved Ones with Dementia." *American Journal of Alzheimer's Disease* (March/April 1998).

Ewing, Wayne. *Tears in God's Bottle: Reflections on Alzheimer's Caregiving.* Tuscon: Whitestone Circle Press, 1999.

Feil, Naomi. *Validation Therapy.* Baltimore: Health Professions Press, 1993.

Filley, Christopher. "Confronting Alzheimer's Disease." *Rocky Mountain Chapter Alzheimer's Association Chapter News,* 16, 4 (autumn 1996).

Frankl, Viktor E. *Man's Search for Meaning.* New York: Pocket Books, 1946.

Greutzer, Howard. *Alzheimer's: A Caregiver's Guide. New York:* Wiley & Sons, Inc., 1992.

Kitwood, Tom. *Dementia Reconsidered.* Reprint. Philadelphia: Open University Press, 1998.

Mace, Nancy L. and Peter B. Rabins. *The 36-Hour Day.* Revised edition. New York: Warner Books, 2000.

Marcell, Jacqueline. *Elder Rage.* 2d ed. Irvine, California: Impressive Press, 2001.

McGowin, Diana Friel. *Living in the Labyrinth.* New York: Dell Publishing, 1993.

Meuser, Thomas M., Ph.D. and Samuel J. Marwit, Ph.D. "A Comprehensive, Stage-Sensitive Model of Grief in Dementia Caregiving." *The Gerontologist* 41, 5 (2001).

Meuser, Thomas M., Ph.D. and Samuel J. Marwit, Ph.D. "Development and Initial Validation of an Inventory to Assess Grief in Caregivers of Persons with Alzheimer's Disease." *The Gerontologist* 42, 6 (2002).

Murphy, Beverly Bigtree. *He Used to Be Somebody.* Boulder, Colorado: Gibbs Associates, 1996.

Nuland, Sherwin. *How We Die.* New York: Vintage, 1995.

Oliver, Rose and Frances A. Bock. *Coping With Alzheimer's: A Caregiver's Emotional Survival Guide.* New York: Wilshire Company, 1991.

Remen, Rachel N., M. D. *Kitchen Table Wisdom.* New York: Riverhead Books, 1996.

Remen, Rachel N., M. D. *My Grandfather's Blessings.* New York: Riverhead Books, 2000.

Rose, Larry. *Show Me the Way to Go Home.* Forest Knolls, California: Elder Books, 1995.

Shenk, David. *The Forgetting.* New York: Doubleday, 2001.

Snowdon, David. *Aging With Grace.* New York: Bantum Doubleday, 2001.

Squires, Sally. "Alzheimer's Burden Heavy on Caregivers." The Washington Post, 6 September 1994.

Tanzi, Rudy and Ann Parsons. *Decoding Darkness.* New York: Perseus Publishers, 2000.

Teichert, Nancy W. "Hopes Rise in War on Alzheimer's." The Sacramento Bee, Online, 30 April 2001. <http://www/sacbee.com/news>

Thoreau, Henry David. *A Year in Thoreau's Journal: 1851.* New York: Penguin Books, 1993.

Waldman, Jackie with Janis L. Dworkis. *The Courage to Give.* Berkley, California: Conari Press, 2000.

Warner, Mark. *Alzheimer's-Proofing Your Home.* 2d ed. West Lafayette, Indiana: Purdue University Press, 2000.

Willard, Nancy. *Telling Time.* New York: Harcourt Brace, 1993.

Internet Sites

Alzheimer's Association. <http://www.alz.org>

Ageless Design. <http://agelessdesign.com/>

Art, Health, Medicine.
   <http://www.cofa.unsw.edu.au/research/stanford/artmed/papers.html>

Gerinet Health Care Discussion Group. e-mail:
   GERINET@UBVM.CC.BUFFALO.EDU

Society For the Arts in Healthcare. <http://www.societyartshealthcare.org/>

The Alzheimer's Page. Gateway to The Alzheimer's List. Sponsored by Washington University's Alzheimer's Disease Research Center, St. Louis. <http://www5.biostat.wustl.edu/alzheimer/>

Time Slips. <http://www.timeslips.org/go.html>

Professional Persons

Carton, Emily. Director, Thetford House Assisted Living Facility, Washington, D.C.

DuBoff, Eugene, M.D. Summit Research, Denver, Colorado.

Garberson, Whit, MSW. Boston, Massachusetts.

Gwyther, Lisa P. ACSW, Duke University.

Hall, Geri. Ph.D., ARNP, FAAN. University of Iowa associate professor, Director of Master's Programs in the College of Nursing, and Advanced Practical Nurse in the Department of Behavioral Neurology, University of Iowa.

Lessard, Janice M.D., FRCP(C). Internist and geriatrician, Toronto, Canada.

McCutcheon, Alan. Staff specialist in geriatric medicine, Department of Community and Geriatric Medicine, Fremantle Hospital, Australia.

Paris, Daniel, MSW. Case Manager, New York, New York.